Dear Alex

It w
meeting you recently in
Phoenix. I hope this book

QUOTES THAT
INSPIRE
WELLBEING

provides you with a few
sparks of motivation and
lots of reasons to laugh
out loud !

Kind regards,

QUOTES THAT INSPIRE WELLBEING

1,000 Sparks of Motivation
to Help You Live Healthy and
Laugh Out Loud!

M. J. White

DEDICATION

*This book is dedicated to my parents,
Jim and Shirley White. Their lifelong
example has inspired in me an
ongoing love for learning and
a desire to continuously improve.*

Contents

ACKNOWLEDGMENTS

Researching inspiring quotes is easy - they are everywhere! However, describing an author in a few sentences is challenging. Wikipedia was most often my go-to source for information. I am very grateful to Wikipedia for the valuable free service that they provide and the positive contribution they make to the world's knowledge base. Many of the authors that I included did not have a Wikipedia entry. In those cases, I utilized search engines and websites to provide background information that I thought would interest the reader and give context to the quote.

Cover design by Ida Fia Sveningsson
(www.idafiasveningsson.se)

Illustrations by Vuong Minh Do
(dovuongminh@gmail.com)

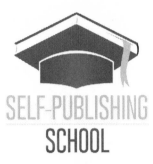

SELF-PUBLISHING
SCHOOL

NOW IT'S YOUR TURN

**Discover the EXACT 3-step blueprint you need
to become a bestselling author in 3 months.**

Self-Publishing School helped me, and now I want
them to help you with this FREE WEBINAR!

Even if you're busy, bad at writing, or don't know where to
start, you CAN write a bestseller and build your best life.

With tools and experience across a variety niches and
professions, Self-Publishing School is the **only** resource
you need to take your book to the finish line!

DON'T WAIT
Watch this FREE WEBINAR now, and
Say "YES" to becoming a bestseller:

INTRODUCTION

Who doesn't love a quote that makes them smile, laugh, or inspires them to be their best self? This book promises to provide that experience 1,000 times! Keep it by your bedside, on a coffee table, at your desk, in your phone, on your computer, or in your purse. Whenever you need a jolt of inspiration or a spark of humor in your life, this book can be your lifeline to a smile!

For years, I collected quotes that I found motivating or encouraging, but I would just write them down and stick them in a file. That all changed when I started working for a fast-growing tech company led by its highly regarded founder and leader. My job was to promote a healthy culture at work. The big boss thought that starting each day off with an inspirational message would assist in that effort. So, I reached into my quote collection and started sharing. People responded very positively, and it dawned on me that this effort could benefit a lot more people. The idea of a book full of healthy, inspiring quotes was born. The project needed a name that accurately described its spirit. After dozens of creative attempts, "**Quotes That Inspire Wellbeing – 1,000 Sparks of Motivation to Help You Live Healthy and Laugh Out Loud!**" fell straight from the heavens onto the cover!

Encouraging optimal health and wellbeing at work is my passion, and I believe that this book of healthy and inspiring quotes can be a helpful and inspirational tool for people at work, at home, or wherever else they may be. The worksite especially can and should be a place where people learn, experiment with, and continuously improve on their lifestyle behaviors. Since adults spend most of their waking hours at work, and because health and safety are reinforced there, it is the natural place for healthy behaviors to be taught, supported, and encouraged. Individuals, families, employers, and society at large all benefit from work environments that help people live healthier, happier and more productive lives. Sprinkle some inspiration and humor in, and you have a formula for a fun and engaging way to raise awareness and promote positive change.

The question is: how? I decided that my contribution to the solution had to contain one thousand knock-your-socks-off quotes specific to maximizing wellbeing - body, mind, and spirit. Some serious research was required to find one thousand of the very best quotes on these topics. I made some rules for myself that included:

- Only two quotes per author (I gave myself a pass and included five of my own)
- At least one-third of the quotes should be, what I call, "healthy humor" - quotes that make smiles appear spontaneously! (they are highlighted with a ☺)
- A diverse set of authors should be represented
- Brief background information on the authors should be provided to add context to the quotes
- Quotes with unknown authors should be limited
- Quotes from thought leaders on health and wellbeing topics should be included

In the end, over 5,000 quotes were collected, categorized, ranked and researched in order to verify authorship and provide background information. The quotes were then divided into the following four categories:

1. Habits
2. The Body
3. The Mind
4. The Spirit

The category on "Habits" was included because healthy habits make achieving health and wellbeing so much easier. Healthy habits make good choices automatic and help us avoid the struggle that comes with having to make a decision. The "Body" category focuses on all aspects of physical wellbeing, including fitness, health, and nutrition. The "Mind" section includes quotes on mental, financial and career-related wellbeing. Finally, the "Spirit" quotes focus on community, emotional, social and spiritual wellbeing. Categories are further divided into sub-categories that address specific topics. The thread tying them all together is the "healthy humor" quotes that are found throughout the book.

Here are my Top 10 ways to use this book for inspiration, learning, and laughs:

1. Sit down with your favorite beverage and read it from cover to cover. Repeat often.
2. Read a quote each morning and night. Consider giving it a personal ranking from 1 to 5, so that you can come back and easily find your favorites and commit them to memory.
3. Share your favorite quotes with friends, or play "Guess Who Said It?" (Author's name? Male or female? Dead or alive? Country of birth? What century is it from?)
4. Choose a famous quote and write down one or two different endings to the quote. Read all the quotes

and have others try to pick the authentic one. Vote on which quote is the best.

5. Good quotes are great for playing the telephone game. Begin with one person selecting a short quote and whispering the quote to the person next to them. Each person does the same until everyone has received the whispered quote. The last person shares what they heard, and then the first person reads the original quote. You never know, the quote you end up with may be just as inspirational as the original. Make it harder by having the listener balance on one leg while being whispered to!

6. Post favorite quotes on a regular basis to your social media sites or include them in texts or emails to share inspiration or laughs.

7. Share a favorite quote each day with family members or colleagues at work. A little dose of inspiration or humor can have a positive effect on everyone in the workplace.

8. Print and post a different quote each day in a high traffic area at home or work that can be seen by everyone who passes by.

9. Dig deeper into the background of authors whose quotes you enjoy. Learn what life experiences might have contributed to their quotations. Find other authors' quotes on similar subjects, or if a quote really touches you, read the work that it came from.

10. Memorize one quote at a time and see how often you can refer to them in conversations.

Please enjoy "**Quotes That Inspire Wellbeing – 1,000 Sparks of Motivation to Help You Live Healthy and Laugh Out Loud!**" Send me your thoughts and any favorite quotes that you would like to see in future books, so that others may be inspired or find a reason to smile – or even laugh out loud!

Follow the "Lean Wellness Blog and Quotes" at www.leanwellness.us

Contact me at mjwhite@leanwellness.us

HABITS

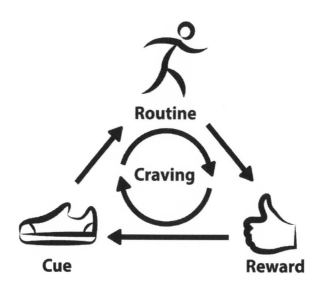

Introduction

Habits? Why include quotes about habits in a book focused on health and wellbeing? The reason is that good habits make living a healthy lifestyle so much easier and enjoyable. Create new habits, or change bad ones, and you're ready to make room in your life for a lot more energy and fun!

Charles Duhigg, in his best-selling book, *The Power of Habit* (2012), describes how habits are formed, how old ones can be changed, and how new ones can be purposefully created. He cites a 2006 Duke research paper that found that more than 40% of our actions are performed out of habit. Duhigg describes habits as, "choices that all of us deliberately make at some point, and then stop thinking about but continue doing, often every day." The author describes it as a process that our brain utilizes to reduce its workload. Once we understand how habit formation works, we can pick and choose which habits to form in our minds.

Duhigg describes habits as a three-step loop that includes: CUE > ROUTINE > REWARD. First, a CUE (or trigger) signals the brain to choose an established habit and go into automatic mode. This is followed by a ROUTINE that can be played out physically, mentally, or emotionally. Lastly, a REWARD is obtained for following the routine, which reinforces the process, or habit loop, in our memory. Over time, this habit loop becomes more and more automatic and leads to the development of a CRAVING for the reward at the end. This subconscious craving becomes the driver of the habit loop.

As an example, if I want to begin a new exercise habit, I might do the following:

Cue: I see my workout clothes laid out when I wake up in the morning.

Routine: I get dressed and engage in 30 minutes of my favorite physical activity.

Reward: I experience happiness when I step on the scale or put on my favorite jeans, and I feel energized all day.

Craving: Every day I find myself desiring and seeking the sense of accomplishment and energy that the routine provides.

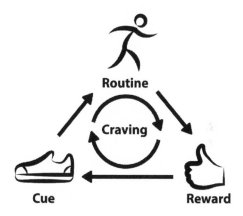

Habits can be purposefully formed, and they can be purposefully changed as well. To change a habit, change the response to a cue. An example might be that noontime is your cue to grab lunch. Using the cue to signal that it's time for something different, a walk for example, can change the habit if you have a suitable reward. This reward will include feel-good endorphins that will keep you alert and energized all afternoon. Over time, the reward will become a craving and the habit will have been totally changed before you know it.

It's easy, decide what behavior you would like to create or change. Then, create a habit loop with a cue, routine, reward, and identify what would make you crave doing it so that really sticks with you. The goal is to create lifestyle behaviors that will become effortless and will add energy to your day and quality to your life.

Habits

1. "Habits are like financial capital – forming one today is an investment that will automatically give out returns for years to come."

   Achor, Shawn – a happiness researcher, author, and speaker who is an expert on positive psychology. He is the author of *The Happiness Advantage* and founder of GoodThink, Inc. (1978-)

2. "Habits are formed by the repetition of particular acts. They are strengthened by an increase in the number of repeated acts. Habits are also weakened or broken, and contrary habits are formed by the repetition of contrary acts."

   Adler, Mortimer – a popular author, philosopher, and educator. (1902-2001)

3. "The best kind of happiness is a habit you're passionate about."

Alder, Shannon – an author of inspirational and uplifting literature.

4. "The law of harvest is to reap more than you sow. Sow an act, and you reap a habit. Sow a habit and you reap a character. Sow a character and you reap a destiny."

Allen, James – a British author. (1864-1912)

5. "Optimal health is a journey taken one step, one habit, and one day at a time."

Andersen, Wayne Scott – a physician, bestselling author, and co-founder of *Take Shape for Life*, which helps people make changes in their lifestyles in order to create optimal health.

6. "We are what we repeatedly do. Excellence, therefore, is not an act but a habit."

Aristotle – an ancient Greek philosopher who is considered to be the first genuine scientist in history. (384-322 BC)

7. "Times of transition are strenuous, but I love them. They are an opportunity to purge, rethink priorities, and be intentional about new habits. We can make our new normal any way we want."

Armstrong, Kristin – a professional road racing cyclist and two-time Olympic gold medalist. (1973-)

8. "The best gifts anyone can give to themselves are good health habits."

> Barrier, Ellen – an author, artist, and musician.

9. "Not managing your time and making excuses are two bad habits. Don't put them both together by claiming you don't have the time."

> Bennett, Bo – a businessman, author, motivational speaker, and amateur comedian. (1972-)

10. ☺ "Old habits are strong and jealous."

> Brande, Dorothea – a writer and editor whose book *Becoming a Writer* (1934) is still in print. She also wrote *Wake Up and Live* (1936), which sold over two million copies and was made into a musical by Twentieth Century Fox in 1937. (1893-1948)

11. "The people you surround yourself with influence your behaviors, so choose friends who have healthy habits."

> Buettner, Dan – *New York Times* bestselling author who became popular with his 2008 book *The Blue Zones: Lessons for Living Longer From the People Who've Lived the Longest*. He is the founder of Blue Zones, LLC and Blue Zones Project - a partnership with the global health and wellbeing company, Sharecare. (1960-)

12. "The awareness that health is dependent upon habits that we control makes us the first generation in history that to a large extent determines its own destiny."

> Carter, Jimmy – the 39th President of the United States who served from 1977-1981. He was a Democrat from rural

Georgia and was a peanut farmer, Georgia State Senator and Governor of Georgia before being elected President. (1924-)

13. ☺ "Curious things, habits. People themselves never knew they had them."

Christie, Agatha – an English crime novelist, short story writer, and playwright. (1890-1976)

14. "Success is the sum of small efforts – repeated day in and day out."

Collier, Robert – an author of self-help and New Thought metaphysical books in the 20th century. (1885-1950)

15. "Depending on what they are, our habits will either make us or break us. We become what we repeatedly do."

Covey, Sean – a motivational speaker and son of bestselling author Stephen Covey. (1964-)

16. "A change in bad habits leads to a change in life."

Craig, Jenny – a weight loss, weight management, and nutrition company founder. The company started in Melbourne, Australia in 1983 and began operations in the United States in 1985. Today, there are more than 700 weight management centers in Australia, the United States, Canada, and New Zealand. (1932-)

17. ☺ "Habits are safer than rules; you don't have to watch them. And you don't have to keep them either. They keep you."

Crane, Frank – a Presbyterian minister, speaker, and columnist. (1861-1928)

18. **"Habits of the mind also provide our mental framework – the way we see the world."**

Dokhampa, Gyalwa – a Buddhist Spiritual master and author of *Restful Mind*. (1981-)

19. **"It seems, in fact, as though the second half of a man's life is made up of nothing, but the habits he has accumulated during the first half."**

Dostoevsky, Fyodor – a Russian novelist and philosopher who wrote about the political, social, and spiritual struggles of Russia in the 1800s. His most famous novels include *Crime and Punishment* (1866) and *The Brothers Karamazov* (1880). (1821-1881)

20. ☺ **"We first make our habits, and then our habits make us."**

Dryden, John – an English poet. (1631-1700)

21. **"Change might not be fast and it isn't always easy. But with time and effort, almost any habit can be reshaped."**

Duhigg, Charles – a *New York Times* reporter and author of *The Power of Habit: Why We Do What We Do in Life* and *Business* (2012) and *Smarter Faster Better - The Secrets of Being Productive in Life and Business* (2016). (1974-)

22. **"A nail is driven out by another nail; habit is overcome by habit."**

Erasmus, Desiderius – a Dutch Catholic priest and social critic during the Dutch Renaissance. He was the first editor of the *New Testament*. (1466-1536)

23. ☺ "Zoo: An excellent place to study the habits of human beings."

Esar, Evan – a humorist who wrote *Esar's Comic Dictionary* (1943), *Humorous English* (1961) and *20,000 Quips and Quotes* (1968). His quotes can often be found in crossword puzzles. (1899-1995)

24. ☺ "My problem lies in reconciling my gross habits with my net income."

Flynn, Errol – an Australian-born actor who achieved Hollywood fame for his romantic swashbuckler roles. (1909-1959)

25. "Design your life to minimize reliance on willpower."

Fogg, B.J. – an expert in behavioral change at Stanford University. His Persuasive Technology Lab focuses on methods for creating habits – first, by showing what causes behavior, then automating behavior change, and finally persuading people via mobile phones.

26. "If you pick the right small behavior and sequence it right, then you won't have to motivate yourself to have it grow. It will just happen naturally, like a good seed planted in a good spot."

Fogg, B.J. – an expert in behavioral change at Stanford University. His Persuasive Technology Lab focuses on methods for creating habits – first, by showing what causes behavior, then automating behavior change, and finally persuading people via mobile phones.

27. "It is easier to prevent bad habits than to break them."

Franklin, Benjamin – a Founding Father of the United States and influential author, politician, scientist, and inventor. (1706-1790)

28. ☺ **"Your net worth to the world is usually determined by what remains after your bad habits are subtracted from your good ones."**

Franklin, Benjamin – a Founding Father of the United States and influential author, politician, scientist, and inventor. (1706-1790)

29. **"Your beliefs become your thoughts, Your thoughts become your words, Your words become your actions, Your actions become your habits, Your habits become your values, Your values become your destiny."**

Gandhi, Mahatma – a political and spiritual figure who led India to independence from British rule through non-violent civil disobedience. Gandhi's approach inspired peaceful movements for civil rights and freedom around the world, including the American civil rights movement of the 1960s. (1869-1948)

30. **"Your little choices become habits that affect the bigger decisions you make in life."**

George, Elizabeth – a bestselling author and national speaker dedicated to helping people live a deeper spiritual life. Her radio broadcast, *A Minute for Busy Women*, is featured on Christian radio stations across the United States and at *www.OnePlace.com*.

31. ☺ **"Habits are where our lives and careers and bodies are made."**

Godin, Seth – an author, entrepreneur, and speaker. His books include: *Purple Cow* (2003), *The Dip* (2007), and *Linchpin: Are You Indispensable?* (2010). (1960-)

32. ☺ **"If you want to get in shape, go to the gym every single day, change your clothes and take a shower. If you can do that every single day for a month, pretty soon you'll start doing something while you're there."**

Godin, Seth – an author, entrepreneur, and speaker. His books include: *Purple Cow* (2003), *The Dip* (2007), and *Linchpin: Are You Indispensable?* (2010). (1960-)

33. **"Your social networks may matter more than your genetic networks. But if your friends have healthy habits you are more likely to as well. So, get healthy friends."**

Hyman, Mark – a physician, bestselling author, and proponent of functional medicine. He serves as chairman of the Institute for Functional Medicine and is the founder and medical director of the UltraWellness Center. His books include: *Food: What the Heck Should I Eat? (2018), Eat Fat, Get Thin (2016), 10-Day Detox Diet (2014),* and *The Blood Sugar Solution (2012).* (1959-)

34. ☺ **"Good habits are worth being fanatical about."**

Irving, John – a novelist and Academy Award-winning screenwriter. He achieved fame for the film *The World According to Garp* (1982). (1942-)

35. **"The chains of habit are too weak to be felt until they are too strong to be broken."**

Johnson, Samuel – an English writer who made a lasting contribution to English literature. (1709-1784)

36. "A man who can't bear to share his habits is a man who needs to quit them."

King, Stephen – an author of horror, supernatural fiction, suspense, science fiction, and fantasy. His 54 novels and six non-fiction books have sold more than 350 million copies. (1947-)

37. "Habits define who we are from the outside in, more than who we are defines us from the inside out."

Kintz, Jarod – author of *This Book Has No Title*. (1982-)

38. "Habit is a cable; we weave a thread each day, and at last we cannot break it."

Mann, Horace – known as the "Father of the Common School Movement." He was a lawyer, politician, and educational reformer who was a leader in establishing universal public education in the United States. (1796-1859)

39. ☺ "It's just like magic. When you live by yourself, all of your annoying habits are gone."

Markoe, Merrill – an author, television writer, and comedian. (1948-)

40. ☺ "Bad Habits are like having a sumo wrestler in the back of your canoe rowing the opposite direction."

Norris, J. Loren – a motivational speaker and television personality who offers lessons on leadership, faith, and family.

41. "Habits change into character."

Ovid – a Roman poet. (43 BC-17 AD)

42. "Nothing is stronger than habit."

Ovid – a Roman poet. (43 BC-17 AD)

43. "Enthusiasm is the electricity of life. How do you get it? You act enthusiastic until you make it a habit."

Parks, Gordon – a prominent photographer and film director who focused on issues of civil rights, poverty, African-Americans, and glamour photography. He was the first African-American to produce and direct major motion pictures. (1912-2006)

44. "If you are going to achieve excellence in big things, you develop the habit in little matters. Excellence is not an exception, it is a prevailing attitude."

Powell, Colin – a retired four-star Army general and the first African-American to serve as Secretary of State. His 35-year military career included serving as Chairman of the Joint Chiefs of Staff. (1937-)

45. "We can never free ourselves from habit. But we can replace bad habits with good ones."

Pressfield, Steven – a successful author of historical fiction, non-fiction, and screenplays. His struggles to earn a living as a writer, including a period of time when he was homeless and living in his car, are described in his 2002 book *The War of Art*. (1943-)

46. "We can use decision–making to choose the habits we want to form, use willpower to get the habit started,

then – and this is the best part – we can allow the extraordinary power of habit to take over. At that point, we're free from the need to decide and the need to use willpower."

Rubin, Gretchen – a bestselling author, blogger and speaker. Her *New York Times* bestsellers include *The Four Tendencies* and #1 bestseller, *The Happiness Project*. She writes on the subjects of habits, happiness, and human nature. (1966-)

47. "Weight loss is a sum of all of your habits - not individual ones."

Ryan, Helen – the author of *21 Days to Change Your Body*. She says, "I am an author, writer, fitness pro, speaker, rock music photographer, mom, and a fierce chocolate lover. Oh, and as I like to say, an 'instigator of change.'"

48. "Motivation is what gets you started. Habit is what keeps you going."

Ryun, Jim – a track and field athlete who won a silver medal during the 1968 Summer Olympics in the 1,500-meter run. He was the first high school athlete to run a mile in under four minutes. (1947-)

49. ☺ "Statistics show that of those who contract the habit of eating, very few survive."

Shaw, George Bernard – an Irish playwright who wrote more than 60 plays and had a major influence on Western culture. He was awarded the Nobel Prize in Literature in 1925. (1856-1950)

50. "Everything you are used to, once done long enough, starts to seem natural, even though it might not be."

Smith, Julien – the Canadian co-founder of Breather, a Montreal-based short-term space rental company. He describes himself as someone who detects patterns and expresses ideas clearly. He has collaborated with recognized thinkers and authored bestselling books.

51. "Laws are never as effective as habits."

Stevenson II, Adlai E. – a lawyer, diplomat, and Democratic politician from Illinois. He was admired for his intellect, speaking ability, and leadership. (1900-1965)

52. ☺ "Why does a woman work ten years to change a man's habits and then complain that he's not the man she married?"

Streisand, Barbra – one of the bestselling musical artists of all time, and the only female and artist outside of rock-n-roll in the Top 10. Her career has lasted more than 60 years, and she is one of only a few entertainers who has been honored with an Emmy, Grammy, Oscar, Tony and a Peabody Award. (1942-)

53. "Creativity is a habit, and the best creativity is the result of good work habits."

Tharp, Twyla – a dancer, choreographer, and author from New York City. In 1966, she formed her own company, Twyla Tharp Dance, which is popular for integrating classical music, jazz, and contemporary pop music. (1941-)

54. ☺ "The habit of reading is the only enjoyment in which there is no alloy; it lasts when all other pleasures fade."

Trollope, Anthony – a popular English novelist during the Victorian era. (1815-1882)

55. ☺ "Bad habits: easy to develop and hard to live with. Good habits: hard to develop and easy to live with."

Woodward, Orrin – the bestselling co-author of *Launching a Leadership Revolution* with Chris Brady and *LeaderShift* with Oliver DeMille. He has also authored *And Justice For All: The Quest for Concord* and *RESOLVED: 13 Resolutions for LIFE*.

THE BODY

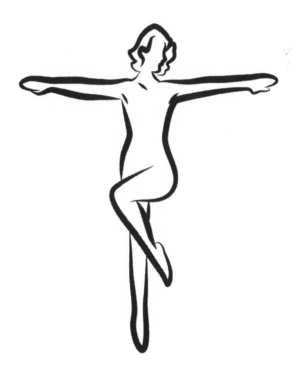

Introduction

Seventy-five percent or more of all that is physically wrong with us is due to chronic (persisting for a long time) health conditions, which are the direct result of lifestyle behaviors. In a nutshell:

- We do not move enough.
- We do not eat or drink healthy food.
- Almost 20 percent of us use tobacco.
- 40 percent of us get less than the recommended amount of sleep.
- The majority of us are overly stressed most of the time.

For more than ten years, I have promoted healthy lifestyle behaviors in all kinds of work environments. Watching people struggle trying to keep up with the latest diet fads and exercise gimmicks, led me to come up with a simple prescription for fixing all that ails us. It's called MEDSS, and it's all you need to know to start improving your health and wellbeing today. The MEDSS prescription for thriving in body, mind, and spirit is based on the following:

- Move more
- Eat and drink healthy
- Do not use tobacco
- Sleep well
- Stress less

Here's how to put it into action:

1. Move more - Make walking part of your daily routine and reduce the amount of time you spend sitting.

2. Eat and drink healthy - Reduce or eliminate sugar-sweetened beverages from your diet and limit alcohol consumption to recommended levels. Make water or unsweetened tea your go-to beverages.
3. Do not use tobacco in any form - enough said.
4. Sleep well - Make at least seven hours of sleep a top priority. Schedule it!
5. Stress less - Just breathe. Clear your thoughts and focus on breathing in and out for at least five minutes at a time.

It's that simple, and it won't cost you any time or money. In fact, your improved health and vitality will give you more of both. So, take your MEDSS every day!

The Body section includes quotes in the following areas:

- Aging, 56-75
- Body & Health, 76-108
- Body-Mind Connection, 109-117
- Exercise & Fitness, 118-186
- Food & Nutrition, 187-270
- Health Care, 271-283
- Healthy Lifestyle, 284-306
- Prevention & Self-care, 307-322
- Sleep, 323-339
- Weight Management, 340-370

Aging

56. ☺ "The secret to staying young is to live honestly, eat slowly, and lie about your age."

Ball, Lucille – a comedian and actress who is best known for her starring role in the television series *I Love Lucy*. (1911-1989)

57. "I think that age as a number is not nearly as important as health. You can be in poor health and be pretty miserable at 40 or 50. If you're in good health, you can enjoy things into your 80s."

Barker, Bob – a former television game show host, best known for *The Price Is Right* - the longest-running daytime game show in American television history. (1923-)

58. ☺ "Life moves pretty fast. If you don't stop and look once in a while, you could miss it."

Bueller, Ferris – a fictional character in the popular 1986 movie *Ferris Bueller's Day Off*.

59. ☺ "If you ask what is the single most important key to longevity, I would have to say it is avoiding worry, stress and tension. And if you didn't ask me, I'd still have to say it."

Burns, George – a comedian and actor who was one of the few entertainers who experienced success over 75 years - spanning vaudeville, radio, movies, and television. He and wife, Gracie Allen, formed the comedy duo of Burns and Allen. In 1977, at age 81, he played the role of God in the hit movie *Oh, God!* (1896-1996)

60. ☺ "I was thinking about how people seem to read the Bible a whole lot more as they get older; then it dawned on me - they're cramming for their final exam."

Carlin, George - an influential stand-up comedian who was also an actor, social critic, and author. His subject matter often focused on controversial topics like politics, psychology, and religion. (1937-2008)

61. ☺ "The body is like a car: the older you become the more care you have to take care of it - and you don't leave a Ferrari out in the sun."

Collins, Joan - an English-born actress, author, and columnist, who was made famous in her role in the popular 1980s show *Dynasty*. She is the sister of author Jackie Collins. (1933-)

62. "Age does not depend upon years, but upon temperament and health. Some men are born old, and some never grow so."

Edwards, Tryon - a theologian who is best known for compiling *A Dictionary of Thoughts*, a book of quotations. (1809-1894)

63. ☺ "For all the advances in medicine, there is still no cure for the common birthday."

Glenn, John - a Marine Colonel, astronaut, and United States senator. He became one of America's first astronauts in 1959. In 1998, at age 77, he became the oldest person to fly in space. He was awarded the Presidential Medal of Freedom in 2012. (1921-2016)

64. ☺ "Men do not quit playing because they grow old; they grow old because they quit playing."

Holmes Jr., Oliver Wendell – a United States Supreme Court Justice from 1902-1932. He is famous for his long service, concise opinions, and respect for the decisions of elected legislatures. He retired at age 90 as the oldest Justice in the Supreme Court's history and remains one of its most cited justices of all time. (1841-1935)

65. ☺ "I can't die, it would ruin my image."

LaLanne, Jack – called the "Godfather of American Fitness," he was an exercise and nutrition expert who hosted *The Jack LaLanne Show* from 1953-1985. In 1974, at age 60, he swam from Alcatraz Island to Fisherman's Wharf in San Francisco, handcuffed and shackled, while towing a 1,000-pound boat! (1914-2011)

66. ☺ "The older I grow the more I distrust the familiar doctrine that age brings wisdom."

Mencken, H. L. – known as the "Sage of Baltimore," he is considered one of the most influential American writers of the first half of the 20th century and was a respected cultural critic and scholar of American English. (1880-1956)

67. "Do you realize that there is nothing in our genes that tells us when to die? There are genetic codes that tell us how to grow, how to breathe, and how to sleep, but NOTHING that tells us to die. So why do we? Because we literally rust and decay our bodies from the inside out with poor food and lifestyle choices."

Michaels, Jillian – a personal trainer, businesswoman, author, and television personality from Los Angeles. She is best known for her appearances on the television show *The Biggest Loser*. (1974-)

68. **"Age is just a number, and agelessness means not buying into the idea that a number determines everything from your state of health to your attractiveness to your value."**

Northrup, Christiane – a practicing OB/GYN physician for 25 years and now a popular writer, speaker, and advocate for women's health and wellness. She teaches women how to thrive throughout life. (1949-)

69. **"My message is "Getting older is inevitable. Aging and deterioration are optional."**

Northrup, Christiane – a practicing OB/GYN physician for 25 years and now a popular writer, speaker, and advocate for women's health and wellness. She teaches women how to thrive throughout life. (1949-)

70. **"Getting older is unavoidable but falling apart is not."**

Ratey, John – a physician, bestselling author, and Harvard Medical School professor. He is a recognized expert in Neuropsychiatry. His book *Spark - The Revolutionary New Science of Exercise and the Brain* established him as a leading authority on the brain-fitness connection. (1948-)

71. ☺ **"It is not how old you are but how you are old."**

Renard, Jules – a French author and philosopher. (1864-1910)

72.   ☺ "It's paradoxical that the idea of living a long life appeals to everyone, but the idea of getting old doesn't appeal to anyone."

Rooney, Andy – a television personality who is most popular for his 33-years on CBS's *60 Minutes*. (1919-2011)

73.   ☺ "There is no cure for birth and death save to enjoy the interval."

Santayana, George – a Spanish-American philosopher, poet, and author. He taught philosophy at Harvard for more than 20 years before resigning and spending the last 40 years of his life writing in Europe. (1863-1952)

74.   ☺ "Just remember, once you're over the hill you begin to pick up speed."

Schopenhauer, Arthur – a German philosopher whose writings on morality and psychology were very influential in the 19th and 20th centuries. He was one of the first Western philosophers to give recognition to Eastern philosophy. (1788-1860)

75.   ☺ "You're never too old to become younger."

West, Mae – an actress, comedian, and Hollywood sex symbol whose career spanned seven decades. (1893-1980)

Body & Health

76. "Health is the thing that makes you feel like that now is the best time of the year."

     Adams, Franklin – a witty newspaper columnist and radio personality. (1881-1960)

77. "Health is the greatest gift, contentment the greatest wealth, faithfulness the best relationship."

     Buddha – the "enlightened one" from northeastern India. He was a spiritual teacher and the founder of Buddhism. (563-483 BC)

78. "Like it or not, in the end, it's one's body. It's literally what carries you through life. There's a reason for the saying, 'If you have your health, you have everything,' and it's true. Old age, disease – these are the great equalizers."

     Bushnell, Candace – an author and columnist who wrote *Sex in the City*. She followed up her bestseller with six more international bestselling novels: *4 Blondes* (2001), *Trading Up* (2003), *Lipstick Jungle* (2005), *One Fifth Avenue* (2008), *The Carrie Diaries* (2010) and *Summer and the City* (2011). (1958-)

79. "Good health is about being able to fully enjoy the time we do have. It is about being as functional as possible throughout our entire lives and avoiding crippling, painful and lengthy battles with disease. There are many better ways to die, and to live."

Campbell, T. Colin – a biochemist featured in the documentary *Forks Over Knives* (2011). He studies the effect of nutrition on long-term health and recommends a low-fat, whole food, plant-based diet. He is the author of the bestselling book on nutrition *The China Study*. (2005).

80. **"He who has health, has hope; and he who has hope, has everything."**

Carlyle, Thomas – a Scottish philosopher, writer, historian, and teacher. He is considered one of the most important social commentators of his time. (1795-1881)

81. **"As a father, physician and nurse, I have a special place in my heart for children, and I know the brief window of opportunity we have to teach them simple lessons that can lead to a lifetime of good health."**

Carmona, Richard – a physician, nurse, police officer, public health administrator, and politician. (1949-)

82. **"He who takes medicine and neglects to diet wastes the skill of his doctors."**

Chinese Proverb

83. **"Some people are willing to pay the price and it's the same with staying healthy or eating healthy. There's some discipline involved. There's some sacrifices."**

Ditka, Mike – the legendary former Chicago Bears player and coach who was especially known for his fiery temper. He led the Bears to a Super Bowl victory in January 1986. (1939-)

84. "I did as much research as I could, and I took ownership of this illness, because if you don't take care of your body, where are you going to live?"

Duffy, Karen – a model, television personality, and actress who was diagnosed with neurosarcoidosis in 1995, a rare incurable disease that attacks the central nervous system. (1962-)

85. "If you don't do what's best for your body, you're the one who comes up on the short end."

Erving, Julius – known as "Dr. J," he is considered one of the best professional basketball players of all-time. From 1971-1987, his leaping ability made him one of the game's most popular players. (1950-)

86. ☺ "Health nuts are going to feel stupid someday, lying in hospitals dying of nothing."

Foxx, Redd – a comedian and actor who is best known for his comedy records and his star role in the 1970's sitcom *Sanford and Son*. (1922-1991)

87. "Health is not valued till sickness comes."

Fuller, Thomas – an English churchman and historian. (1608-1661)

88. "When you are young and healthy, it never occurs to you that in a single second your whole life could change."

Funicello, Annette – an actress and singer who was best known as one of the "Mouseketeers" on the original *Mickey Mouse Club* television show. She was diagnosed with multiple sclerosis in 1992 and died of complications from the disease in 2013. (1942-2013)

89. ☺ "Life - and I don't suppose I'm the first to make this comparison - is a disease: sexually transmitted, and invariably fatal."

Gaiman, Neil – an English author of short fiction, novels, comic books, graphic novels, and films. (1960-)

90. "We need to create a culture where hand-washing is the thing to do, ... If we can just wash our hands, we will have an impact on some of the most common problems, as well as some of the most serious health problems we face."

Gerberding, Julie – a physician, infectious disease expert, and former director of the United States Centers for Disease Control and Prevention (CDC). (1955-)

91. ☺ "Ignore your health and it will go away."

Google Images: Healthy Snack Quotes

92. "Good health is often a matter of good judgment."

Hanks, Marion – a general authority of The Church of Jesus Christ of Latter-day Saints (LDS Church) from 1953 until his death in 2011. (1921-2011)

93. "The root of all health is in the brain. The trunk of it is in emotion. The branches and leaves are the body. The flower of health blooms when all parts work together."

Kurdish Saying

94. ☺ "People always come up to me and say that my smoking is bothering them... Well, it's killing me!"

Liebman, Wendy – a stand-up comedian who shares observational comedy. (1961-)

95. **"The greatest miracle on Earth is the human body. It is stronger and wiser than you may realize and improving its ability to self-heal is within your control."**

Mancini, Fabrizio – a popular chiropractor, author, radio host, and healthy living expert. His books include *The Power of Self-Healing* and *Chicken Soup for the Chiropractic Soul*.

96. ☺ **"So many people spend their health gaining wealth, and then have to spend their wealth to regain their health."**

Materi, A. J. Reb – an employee of the Roman Catholic Diocese of Saskatoon, British Columbia, Canada.

97. **"We're in a situation now where weight and extreme weight and heart disease is the biggest killer in this country today."**

Oliver, Jamie – a British celebrity chef and restaurateur who is known throughout the world for supporting philanthropic causes. (1975-)

98. ☺ **"Quit worrying about your health. It will go away."**

Orben, Robert – a comedy writer who also worked as a magician and a speechwriter for United States President Gerald Ford. (1927-)

99. **"The greatest wealth is health."**

Virgil – an ancient Roman poet who wrote three of the most famous poems in Latin literature: the *Eclogues*, the *Georgics*, and the *Aeneid*. (70-19 BC)

100. "You can't legislate or litigate good, healthy behavior but we must be willing to educate people at an early age about the effects of unhealthy living."

Wamp, Zack – a former Republican Congressman from Tennessee who served from 1995-2011. (1957-)

101. "Improper breathing is a common cause of ill health. If I had to limit my advice on healthier living to just one tip, it would be simply to learn how to breathe correctly. There is no single more powerful – or more simple – daily practice to further your health and wellbeing than breathwork."

Weil, Andrew – a physician and bestselling author on holistic health. He played a major role in establishing integrative medicine, which combines alternative medicine, conventional evidence-based medicine, and other practices into a system that addresses holistic human healing. (1942-)

102. ☺ "A man's health can be judged by which he takes two at a time – pills or stairs."

Welsh, Joan – attributed to Joan Welsh.

103. "Health is a large word. It embraces not the body only, but the mind and spirit as well; and not today's pain or pleasure alone, but the whole being and outlook of a man."

West, James – a Georgia physician whose approach to wellness includes not just helping to heal illness and disease but helping to predict and minimize future challenges to physical and mental wellbeing.

104. ☺ **"Your health is in your hands. Keep them clean."**

White, M. J. – a worksite health promotion professional, writer, and speaker. He is the creator of Lean Wellness – an approach to transforming lifestyle behaviors at work through continuous improvement in body, mind, and spirit. (1957-)

105. **"Your health is what you make of it. Everything you do and think either adds to the vitality, energy and spirit you possess or takes away from it."**

Wigmore, Ann – a Lithuanian-American holistic health practitioner, nutritionist, and author. (1909-1993)

106. **"Health requires healthy food."**

Williams, Roger – a pioneer in Biochemistry and Nutrition who spent his career at the University of Texas at Austin. He played a major role in nutritional research and discovery and wrote about the importance of good nutrition. (1893-1988)

107. **"Health is a state of complete physical, mental and social wellbeing, and not merely the absence of disease or infirmity."**

World Health Organization statement made in 1948.

108. **"Health is the greatest of God's gifts, but we take it for granted; yet it hangs on a thread as fine as a spider's web and the tiniest thing can make it snap, leaving the strongest of us helpless in an instant."**

Worth, Jennifer – a British nurse, musician, and author who wrote a bestselling trilogy about her work as a midwife in a poverty-stricken area of London in the 1950s. A television series based on her books, *Call the Midwife*, started airing on the BBC in 2012. (1935-2011)

Body & Mind Connection

109. **"Don't give up what you want most for what you want now."**

Brinkman, Curt – a wheelchair athlete and motivational speaker. He won the 1980 Boston Marathon's Men's Wheelchair Division and became the first athlete in the wheelchair division to finish in a faster time than the fastest runner. (1953-2010)

110. **"The body says what words cannot."**

Graham, Martha – a modern dancer and choreographer for over 70 years. She is considered to have had more influence on modern dance than anyone else in history. (1894-1991)

111. **"Health is a state of complete harmony of the body, mind and spirit. When one is free from physical disabilities and mental distractions, the gates of the soul open."**

Iyengar, B.K.S. – one of the world's leading yoga teachers. (1918-2014)

112. **"True health can be expressed when there is integration of all aspects of a person's being; physical, mental, emotional, and spiritual."**

Mayo Clinic Health System

113. **"All truly great thoughts are conceived by walking."**

Nietzsche, Friedrich – a German philosopher, cultural critic, poet, and scholar whose work has exerted a profound influence on Western philosophy and modern intellectual history. (1844-1900)

114. **"Our bodies are our gardens—our wills are our gardeners."**

Shakespeare, William – an English poet and playwright who is considered the greatest writer and dramatist in the English language. He wrote approximately 38 plays, among them: *Hamlet, Macbeth, Julius Caesar, The Tempest, Henry IV, King Lear*, and *Romeo and Juliet.* (1564-1616)

115. **"It is no more necessary that a man should remember the different dinners and suppers which have made him healthy, than the different books which have made him wise. Let us see the results of good food in a strong body, and the results of great reading in a full and powerful mind."**

Smith, Sydney – an English writer and Anglican cleric. (1771-1845)

116. **"A healthy outside starts from the inside."**

Ulrich, Robert – an actor who starred in 15 television series during his 30-year career. In 1996, he was diagnosed with a rare form of cancer and sought treatment for his illness while working and raising money for cancer research. After a three-year remission, his cancer returned. He died in 2002 at the age of 55. (1946-2002)

117. "True enjoyment comes from activity of the mind and exercise of the body; the two are united."

> von Humboldt, Alexander – a Prussian explorer and philosopher. (1769-1859)

Exercise & Fitness

118. ☺ "It took me seventeen years to get three thousand hits in baseball. I did it in one afternoon on the golf course."

> Aaron, Hank – a Major League baseball player who held the record for career home runs for 33 years (before the steroid era). The *Sporting News* ranked Aaron fifth on its list of "100 Greatest Baseball Players." (1934-)

119. ☺ "The longest journey begins with a single step, not with a turn of the ignition key."

> Abbey, Edward – an author known for his advocacy of environmental issues, criticism of public land policies, and anarchist political views. (1927-1989)

120. ☺ "If it weren't for the fact that the TV set and the refrigerator are so far apart, some of us wouldn't get any exercise at all."

> Adams, Joey – a comedian whose career lasted more than 70 years. He wrote the *Strictly for Laughs* column in the *New York Post* for many years, hosted his own radio show, and wrote 23 books. He is credited with being the first person to say, "With friends like that, who needs enemies?" (1911-1999)

121. ☺ "I like long walks, especially when they're taken by people who annoy me."

   Allen, Fred – one of the most admired and listened to comedians on the radio. He was often censored for his unacceptable content, but his style and technique had a lasting influence on comedians who came after him. (1894-1956)

122. "If you stretch correctly and regularly, you will find that every movement you make becomes easier."

   Anderson, Bob – a British Olympic fencer and famous choreographer of Hollywood sword fights. (1922-2012)

123. "Wholesome exercise in the free air, under the wide sky, is the best medicine for body and spirit."

   Arnold, Sarah – a school superintendent in Minneapolis and Boston, who was also a school textbook writer. Her elementary textbooks were very popular during the early 20th century. She also served as president of the American Home Economics Association and the Girl Scouts of America. (1859-1943)

124. ☺ "Aerobics: a series of strenuous exercises, which help convert fats, sugars, and starches into aches, pains, and cramps."

   Author Unknown

125. ☺ "I consider my refusal to go to the gym today as resistance training."

   Author Unknown

126. ☺ "Would you rather be covered in sweat at the gym or covered in clothes at the beach?"

Author Unknown

127. ☺ "Smiling is my favorite exercise."

Author Unknown

128. ☺ "There are short-cuts to happiness, and dancing is one of them."

Baum, Vicki – an Austrian-born author who is considered to be one of the first modern bestselling authors. Her books are among the first examples of contemporary mainstream literature. (1888-1960)

129. ☺ "There are really only two requirements when it comes to exercise. One is that you do it. The other is that you continue to do it."

Brand-Miller, J., Foster-Powell, K., Colagiuri, S., and Barclay, A. – from the book *The New Glucose Revolution for Diabetes*.

130. ☺ "The one thing that can solve most of our problems is dancing."

Brown, James – a singer, songwriter, organist, and bandleader who was known as "The Godfather of Soul" and most famous for his electrifying dance moves. He was a major figure in music in the Twentieth Century, with a career that stretched over 60 years and influenced several music genres. (1933-2006)

131. "Strength training, particularly in conjunction with regular aerobic exercise, can also have a profound impact on a person's mental and emotional health."

> Centers for Disease Control and Prevention (CDC) – the leading national public health institute in the United States.

132. ☺ "Fitness – if it came in a bottle, everybody would have a great body."

> Cher – a superstar singer and actress who got her start in the duo *Sonny and Cher* in the 1960s. She won fame with top music hits and movie roles. Her role in the 1987 film *Moonstruck* won her an Oscar for Best Actress. (1946-)

133. "Walking is magic. Can't recommend it highly enough. I read that Plato and Aristotle did much of their brilliant thinking together while ambulating. The movement, the meditation, the health of the blood pumping, and the rhythm of footsteps...this is a primal way to connect with one's deeper self."

> Cole, Paula – a singer-songwriter whose single, *Where Have All the Cowboys Gone?* was a hit in 1997. (1968-)

134. ☺ "If you think lifting weights is dangerous, try being weak. Being weak is dangerous."

> Contreras, Bret – a fitness trainer, speaker, author, and inventor, who is known as "The Glute Guy."

135. ☺ "The wisdom of age: don't stop walking."

> Cooley, Mason – a professor of French, Speech, and World Literature at the College of Staten Island who was known for his witty sayings. (1927-2002)

136. ☺ "Everyone should walk the dog twice a day, whether they have one or not."

> Cooper, Kenneth – a physician, author, and creator of aerobics. The former Air Force Colonel authored the 1968 book *Aerobics* and the popular *The New Aerobics* a few years later. Over 30 million copies of his 18 published books have been sold and have been translated into 41 languages. (1931-)

137. ☺ "We do not stop exercising because we grow old – we grow old because we stop exercising."

> Cooper, Kenneth – a physician, author, and creator of aerobics. The former Air Force Colonel authored the 1968 book *Aerobics* and the popular *The New Aerobics* a few years later. Over 30 million copies of his 18 published books have been sold and have been translated into 41 languages. (1931-)

138. "Exercise is good for your mind, body, and soul."

> Cortright, Susie – an author of several books and founder of *Momscape.com*, a website that helps busy women find balance in their lives.

139. ☺ "Hearty laughter is a good way to jog internally without having to go outdoors."

> Cousins, Norman – a political journalist and author. (1915-1990)

140. "Exercise invigorates the body and sharpens the mind."

> Crichton, Michael – a bestselling author, physician, producer, director, and screenwriter who has had many

of his science fiction, medical fiction, and thriller books turned into movies. (1942-2008)

141. ☺ "I really don't think I need buns of steel. I'd be happy with buns of cinnamon."

DeGeneres, Ellen – recognized simply as "Ellen," she is a very popular talk show host, comedian, writer, and producer. She has been the host of the *Ellen DeGeneres Show* since 2003. (1958-)

142. ☺ "You have to stay in shape. My grandmother, she started walking five miles a day when she was sixty. She's ninety-seven now, and we don't know where the hell she is."

DeGeneres, Ellen – recognized simply as "Ellen," she is a very popular talk show host, comedian, writer, and producer. She has been the host of the *Ellen DeGeneres Show* since 2003. (1958-)

143. ☺ "My idea of exercise is a good brisk sit."

Diller, Phyllis – a stand-up comedian and television personality. (1917-2012)

144. ☺ "I have to exercise in the morning, before my brain figures out what I'm doing."

Doble, Marsha – attributed to Marsha Doble

145. "Typically, people who exercise, start eating better and becoming more productive at work. They smoke less and show more patience with colleagues and family. They use their credit cards less frequently and

say they feel less stressed. Exercise is a keystone habit that triggers widespread change."

Duhigg, Charles – a *New York Times* reporter and author of *The Power of Habit: Why We Do What We Do in Life and Business* (2012) and *Smarter Faster Better - The Secrets of Being Productive in Life and Business* (2016). (1974-)

146. "The human body is made up of some four hundred muscles; evolved through centuries of physical activity. Unless they are used, they will deteriorate."

Fisk, Eugene – a physician, public health advocate, and author. (1867-1931)

147. ☺ "Doctor to patient: "What fits your busy schedule better, exercising one-hour a day or being dead 24 hours a day?"

Glasbergen, Randy – a cartoonist and humorous illustrator who enjoyed three decades of newspaper syndication. (1957-2015)

148. "Muscles are in a most intimate and peculiar sense the organs of the will."

Hall, G. Stanley – a pioneer of child and educational psychology. He was the first American to receive a Ph.D. in psychology. He taught at Johns Hopkins University and was a founder of Clark University. His ideas influenced Sigmund Freud and Charles Darwin. (1846-1924)

149. "Exercise to stimulate, not to annihilate. The world wasn't formed in a day, and neither were we. Set small goals and build upon them."

Haney, Lee – a professional bodybuilder and eight-time winner of the *Mr. Olympia* title. (1959-)

150. **"Resistance training is the only type of exercise that can slow, and even reverse, declines in muscle mass, bone density, and strength that were once considered inevitable results of aging."**

Harvard Health Letter

151. **"Walking is man's best medicine."**

Hippocrates – a Greek physician who is known as the "Father of Modern Medicine." (460-370 BC)

152. ☺ **"Whenever I feel like exercise, I lie down until the feeling passes."**

Hutchins, Robert – an educational philosopher, dean of Yale Law School, and chancellor of the University of Chicago. He was married to novelist Maude Hutchins. (1899-1977)

153. ☺**"Exercise relieves stress. Nothing relieves exercise."**

Ikkaku, Takayuki – a Japanese video game developer at Nintendo who has been developing popular games since 2004, including *Splatoon 2* in 2018.

154. **"As dismaying as it is, shrinking muscles are more than a vanity issue. Diminished strength equals a decreased quality of life. Minus strength, everything is more difficult: Doing chores, going for walks – simply living life to its fullest becomes a challenge."**

Kuzma, Cindy – a freelance health and fitness writer with more than 15 years of experience. She earned her master's degree from Northwestern University and now lives, writes and runs in Chicago. Her work appears in *Men's Health*, *Women's Health* and *Runner's World*.

155. ☺ **"Exercise is king. Nutrition is queen. Put them together and you've got a kingdom."**

LaLanne, Jack – called the "Godfather of American Fitness," he was an exercise and nutrition expert who hosted *The Jack LaLanne Show* from 1953-1985. In 1974, at age 60, he swam from Alcatraz Island to Fisherman's Wharf in San Francisco, handcuffed and shackled, while towing a 1,000-pound boat! (1914-2011)

156. ☺ **"I can't believe anyone would voluntarily run 26 miles. Sometimes I sit on the couch cross-legged because I don't feel like walking to the bathroom."**

Lancaster, Jen – an author of eight memoirs and four novels. After being laid off in 2001, she launched a website and blog, *jennsylvania.com*, to air her frustrations about being unemployed. Her memoir, *The Tao of Martha*, was optioned for a sitcom by FOX. (1967-)

157. ☺ **"A bear, however hard he tries, grows tubby without exercise."**

Milne, A.A. – an English author of books and poems for children who is best known for his books about Winnie-the-Pooh. (1882-1956)

158. ☺ **"Dancing is like dreaming with your feet!"**

Mozart, Constanze – the wife of Wolfgang Amadeus Mozart. Following Mozart's death, she married a writer and together they co-wrote a biography of Mozart. (1762-1842)

159. ☺ "Restore human legs as a means of travel. Pedestrians rely on food for fuel and need no special parking facilities."

Mumford, Lewis – a historian, sociologist, philosopher of technology, and literary critic. He was known for his study of cities and urban architecture. (1895-1990)

160. "Believe it or not, having a really hearty chuckle can help too. This is because laughing gets the diaphragm moving and this plays a vital part in moving blood around the body."

Nelson, Andrea – a lead researcher at the University of Leeds School of Healthcare.

161. "From the top of our heads to the bottom of our toes, physical activity is the stimulus that gets almost all our organs working at their best."

Nelson, Miriam – a professor and researcher at Tufts University. She has published numerous bestsellers and her research led to the creation of the *StrongWomen Program*, a community-based nutrition and exercise program for middle age and older women that operates in over 35 states. (1960-)

162. "We've yet to find a disease where exercise isn't helpful."

Nelson, Miriam – a professor and researcher at Tufts University. She has published numerous bestsellers and her research led to the creation of the *StrongWomen Program*, a community-based nutrition and exercise program for middle age and older women that operates in over 35 states. (1960-)

163. ☺ "The reason they call it 'golf' is that all the other 4 letter words were used up."

   Nielsen, Leslie – a Canadian-American actor and comedian who appeared in more than 100 films and over 150 television programs. (1926-2010)

164. ☺ "Running's a pain in the ass. But, it sure gives me a nice one!"

   Nike Ad

165. ☺ "Wow, I really regret that workout!"

   No one, ever.

166. "The only valid excuse for not exercising is paralysis."

   Nordholt, Moira – a vegan chef, author of *Feel Good Fast*, and owner of the "Feel Good Guru," a vegan takeout restaurant in Toronto. She has been sharing her healthy plant-powered food since 1994.

167. "From an evolutionary perspective, exercise tricks the brain into trying to maintain itself for survival despite the hormonal cues that it is aging."

   Ratey, John – a physician, bestselling author, and Harvard Medical School professor. He is a recognized expert in Neuropsychiatry. His book *Spark - The Revolutionary New Science of Exercise and the Brain* established him as a leading authority on the brain-fitness connection. (1948-)

168. "Eat less, exercise more."

   Rudolph, M. L. – a British-American author who has worked for CNN, HBO, and other television companies around the globe.

169. ☺ "Exercise is a dirty word. Every time I hear it I wash my mouth out with chocolate."

Schulz, Charles – a cartoonist best known for the comic strip *Peanuts*. (1922-2000)

170. ☺ "It's simple, if it jiggles, it's fat."

Schwarzenegger, Arnold – an Austrian-American professional bodybuilder who won the Mr. Olympia contest seven times between 1970-1980. He turned his bodybuilding success into an acting career and is most famous for his *Terminator* character. He also served as Governor of California from 2003-2011. (1947-)

171. ☺ "A fit, healthy body – that is the best fashion statement."

Scott, Jess – a Singapore-born writer who describes herself as an "author/artist/non- conformist." She writes in a variety of non-traditional genres. (1986-)

172. ☺ "Exercise is done against one's wishes and maintained only because the alternative is worse."

Sheehan, George – a physician, author, and senior athlete who is best known for his writing about running. His book *Running & Being: The Total Experience* was a *New York Times* bestseller. (1918-1993)

173. "Walking is the great adventure, the first meditation, a practice of heartiness and soul primary to humankind. Walking is the exact balance between spirit and humility."

Snyder, Gary – a poet, essayist, lecturer, and environmental activist who is associated with the Beat Generation in San

Francisco. He won a Pulitzer Prize for Poetry in 1975 and the American Book Award in 1984. His work is influenced by Buddhist spirituality and nature. (1930-)

174. **"Those who think they have not time for bodily exercise will sooner or later have to find time for illness."**

Stanley, Edward – a British statesman who served as Secretary of State for Foreign Affairs between 1866-1878. His family was one of the richest landowning families in England and his father served as Prime Minister three times. (1826-1893)

175. **"The medical literature tells us that the most effective ways to reduce the risk of heart disease, cancer, stroke, diabetes, Alzheimer's, and many more problems are through healthy diet and exercise. Our bodies have evolved to move, yet we now use the energy in oil instead of muscles to do our work."**

Suzuki, David – a Canadian environmental activist and professor from 1963-2001. He is best known for his television and radio programs, books about nature and the environment, and for criticizing governments for their lack of environmental protection efforts. (1936-)

176. ☺ **"Exercise is for people who can't handle drugs or alcohol."**

Tomlin, Lily – an actress who began her career as a stand-up comedian. Her breakout role was on *Rowan & Martin's Laugh-In*, which she worked on from 1970-1973. (1939-)

177. **"Exercise not only tones the muscles, but also refines the brain and revives the soul."**

    Treanor, Michael – a practicing psychologist in Los Angeles who was a former child actor and martial artist. In the early 1990s, he starred in *3 Ninjas* and *3 Ninjas Knuckle Up*. (1979-)

178. **"Exercise should be regarded as tribute to the heart."**

    Tunney, Gene – the undefeated heavyweight boxing champion from 1926-1928, and light heavyweight champion from 1922-1923. He is considered one of the best technical fighters in boxing history. His title fight with Jack Dempsey, known as "The Long Count Fight," is one of the sport's most famous contests. (1897-1978)

179. **"To enjoy the glow of good health, you must exercise."**

    Tunney, Gene – the undefeated heavyweight boxing champion from 1926-1928, and light heavyweight champion from 1922-1923. He is considered one of the best technical fighters in boxing history. His title fight with Jack Dempsey, known as "The Long Count Fight," is one of the sport's most famous contests. (1897-1978)

180. ☺ **"I am pushing sixty. That is enough exercise for me."**

    Twain, Mark – perhaps America's most famous author and humorist. He is best known for his books *Tom Sawyer* and *Huckleberry Finn*. (1835-1910)

181. ☺ **"Muscles come and go; flab lasts."**

    Vaughan, Bill – a *Kansas City Star* columnist and author. (1915-1977)

182. "Movement is a medicine for creating change in a person's physical, emotional, and mental states."

Welch, Carol – attributed to Carol Welch.

183. ☺ "Hard bodies come with resistance."

White, M. J. – a worksite health promotion professional, writer, and speaker. He is the creator of Lean Wellness – an approach to transforming lifestyle behaviors at work through continuous improvement in body, mind, and spirit. (1957-)

184. ☺ "Workout: short intervals of exercise completed while gazing at a smartphone."

White, M. J. – a worksite health promotion professional, writer, and speaker. He is the creator of Lean Wellness – an approach to transforming lifestyle behaviors at work through continuous improvement in body, mind, and spirit. (1957-)

185. "A vigorous five-mile walk will do more good for an unhappy but otherwise healthy adult than all the medicine and psychology in the world."

White, Paul – a physician and cardiologist who was a leading promoter of preventive medicine. (1886-1973)

186. ☺ "Everywhere is within walking distance if you have the time."

Wright, Steven – a stand-up comedian, actor, writer, and an Oscar-winning film producer. Comedy Central ranked him 23rd in their list of the "Top 100 Greatest Stand-up Comics." (1955-)

Food & Nutrition

187. "There are around 5,000 farmers in the U.S. who still grow tobacco. Every day they work in the fields growing, tending and harvesting the tobacco leaves used to produce cigarettes. Their daily efforts produce a product that kills five million people every year. Despite the evidence against tobacco use, they do it for one reason...the money."

Aldana, Steven – a foremost expert on healthy living and worksite wellness. The quote is from his book *Culture Clash - How We Win The Battle for Better Health.* (2013)

188. "Nobody had ever told me junk food was bad for me. Four years of medical school, and four years of internship and residency, and I never thought anything was wrong with eating sweet rolls and doughnuts, and potatoes, and bread, and sweets."

Atkins, Robert – a cardiologist who is best known for creating the popular and controversial *Atkins Diet,* which emphasizes protein and fat as the primary sources of dietary calories. (1930-2003)

189. ☺ "Your body is a temple, not a drive-through."

Author Unknown

190. "Eat foods that nourish your body and mind. Take time to look at what you're putting in your body and how it's affecting your energy, mood and health. Decide where you could use some improvement and

look into foods and supplements that promote health in that area."

AwesomeLifeTips.com

191. "Man seeks to change the foods available in nature to suit his tastes, thereby putting an end to the very essence of life contained in them."

> Baba, Sai – an Indian spiritual master who was regarded by his followers as a saint, fakir, and Satguru, according to their individual beliefs. (1835-1918)

192. ☺ "Food, like your money, should be working for you!"

> Beckford, Rita – a physician who has maintained an 80 lb. weight loss and is the author of a weight-loss manual for families, *The Beckford Formula, Lose the Fat for Good!* She is also the creator and host of *Home With Dr. B,* a fitness and weight-loss video for beginners.

193. "...we are an overfed and undernourished nation digging an early grave with our teeth..."

> Benson, Ezra – a farmer, government official, and religious leader who served two terms as United States Secretary of Agriculture and as the 13th president of The Church of Jesus Christ of Latter-day Saints. (1899-1994)

194. "It's never too late to start eating well. A good diet can reverse many of those conditions as well. In short: change the way you eat, and you can transform your health for the better."

> Campbell, T. Colin – a biochemist who is featured in the documentary *Forks Over Knives* (2011). He studies the

effect of nutrition on long-term health and recommends a low-fat, whole food, plant-based diet. He is the author of the bestselling book on nutrition *The China Study*. (2005).

195. **"Eating crappy food isn't a reward – it's a punishment."**

Carey, Drew – an actor, comedian, sports executive, and game show host. (1958-)

196. **"The more you eat, the less flavor; the less you eat, the more flavor."**

Chinese Proverb

197. **"Thou should eat to live, not live to eat."**

Cicero, Marcus Tullius – a Roman philosopher and politician who is considered one of Rome's greatest orators and prose writers. (106-43 BC)

198. **"I believe that parents need to make nutrition education a priority in their home environment. It's crucial for good health and longevity to instill in your children sound eating habits from an early age."**

Cora, Cat – a professional chef who is best known for her featured role as an Iron Chef on the Food Network television show *Iron Chef America*. (1967-)

199. **"Purchase items that can be made into several meals, like a whole roasted chicken, or bag of sweet potatoes, and shop the periphery of the grocery store, avoiding the middle aisles full of processed and higher-priced foods."**

Cora, Cat – a professional chef who is best known for

her featured role as an Iron Chef on the Food Network television show *Iron Chef America*. (1967-)

200. **"We are indeed much more than what we eat, but what we eat can nevertheless help us to be much more than what we are."**

Davis, Adelle – a popular nutrition author in the early to mid-1900s who helped influence American eating habits by promoting better health through nutrition. Her writing included a textbook on nutrition (1942) and four bestselling books for consumers. (1904-1974)

201. ☺ **"Eat breakfast like a king, lunch like a prince, and dinner like a pauper."**

Davis, Adelle – a popular nutrition author in the early to mid-1900s who helped influence American eating habits by promoting better health through nutrition. Her writing included a textbook on nutrition (1942) and four bestselling books for consumers. (1904-1974)

202. ☺ **"Vegetables are a must on a diet. I suggest carrot cake, zucchini bread, and pumpkin pie."**

Davis, Jim – a cartoonist who is best known as the creator of the comic strip *Garfield*, which has been published since 1978 and is the world's most widely syndicated comic strip. (1945-)

203. **"The commonest form of malnutrition in the western world is obesity."**

Deitel, Mervyn – a pioneer in bariatric surgery at St. Joseph's Hospital in Toronto from 1971-1996. He was also a founder of the American Society for Bariatric Surgery. (1936-)

204. ☺ "Forget love – I'd rather fall in chocolate!"

Dykes, Sandra – attributed to Sandra J. Dykes.

205. "If you eat a lot of starchy foods, introduce a vegetable once a week, then twice a week, and then three times a week. Slowly fill your diet with new flavors. By the time you're ready to let go of whatever it is you want to let go of, you've got a full menu."

Edelstein, Lisa – an actress and playwright. (1966-)

206. ☺ "If we're not willing to settle for junk living, we certainly shouldn't settle for junk food."

Edwards, Sally – a bestselling author, professional triathlete, and iPhone app developer. She assisted in the development of the Olympic sport of triathlon. (1947-)

207. ☺ "We think fast food is equivalent to pornography, nutritionally speaking."

Elbert, Steve – attributed to Steve Elbert.

208. "All the pre-made sauces in a jar, and frozen and canned vegetables, processed meats, and cheeses which are loaded with artificial ingredients and sodium can get in the way of a healthy diet. My number one advice is to eat fresh, and seasonally."

English, Todd – a celebrity chef, restauranteur, author, entrepreneur and television personality who is based in Boston. (1960-)

209. "The first thing I would do for anyone who's trying to lose body fat, for instance, would be to remove foods from the house that he or she would consume during lapses of self-control."

Ferriss, Tim – an entrepreneur and author of the self-help bestsellers *The 4-Hour Workweek*, *The 4-Hour Body*, and *The 4-Hour Chef*. His podcast is the #1 business podcast on iTunes. (1977-)

210. ☺ "The cucumber and the tomato are both fruit; the avocado is a nut. To assist with the dietary requirements of vegetarians, on the first Tuesday of the month a chicken is officially a vegetable."

Fforde, Jasper – a British novelist whose first novel *The Eyre Affair* was published in 2001. (1961-)

211. "Go vegetable heavy. Reverse the psychology of your plate by making meat the side dish and vegetables the main course."

Flay, Bobby – a celebrity chef, restaurateur, and reality television personality. (1964-)

212. ☺ "Your diet is a bank account. Good food choices are good investments."

Frankel, Bethenny – a television personality, talk show host, author, and entrepreneur. (1970-)

213. "When you gradually add in nutrient-dense, fiber-rich foods, you simply stop feeling cravings. You run out of space in your belly for the old junk. Instead of craving, you feel full, fulfilled, and content."

Freston, Kathy – a self-help author of books on veganism and contributor to the *Huffington Post*.

214. "You know you are addicted to a food if despite knowing it is bad for you and despite wanting to change, you still keep eating it. Addiction means that a craving has more control over your behavior than you do."

Freston, Kathy – a self-help author of books on veganism and contributor to the *Huffington Post*.

215. "Blueberries, strawberries and blackberries are true super foods. Naturally sweet and juicy, berries are low in sugar and high in nutrients – they are among the best foods you can eat."

Fuhrman, Joel – a family physician who specializes in nutrition-based treatments for obesity and chronic disease. (1953-)

216. "We need to take vegetables out of the role of side dish, even in vegetarian diets, whose calories are generally derived mainly from grains and other starches."

Fuhrman, Joel – a family physician who specializes in nutrition-based treatments for obesity and chronic disease. (1953-)

217. ☺ "And there never was an apple, in Adam's opinion, that wasn't worth the trouble you got into for eating it."

Gaiman, Neil – an English author of short fiction, novels, comic books, graphic novels, and films. (1960-)

218. **"More die in the United States of too much food than of too little."**

Galbraith, John Kenneth – a widely respected Canadian-American economist, public official, and diplomat. He taught economics at Harvard for 50 years and was a prolific author and writer on a variety of subjects. (1908-2006)

219. **"With the chronic obesity in America, it's more important than ever to not only feed kids healthy foods but to teach them how to make healthy choices on their own."**

Garth, Jennie – an actress and film director. (1972-)

220. ☺**"Don't eat anything with more than five ingredients, or ingredients you can't pronounce."**

Google Images: Healthy Snack Quotes

221. ☺ **"If we're not supposed to have midnight snacks, then why is there a light in the fridge?"**

Google Images: Healthy Snack Quotes

222. ☺ **"You are what you eat, so don't be fast, cheap, easy or fake."**

Google Images: Healthy Snack Quotes

223. ☺ **"As a child my family's menu consisted of two choices: take it or leave it."**

Hackett, Buddy – a comedian and actor. (1924-2003)

224. "With all of the holiday cheer in the air, it's easy to overlook the ingredients in the foods. Ingredients such as salt, sugar, and fat - all of which leads to diseases such as high blood pressure, diabetes, strokes, heart disease, and cancer."

Haney, Lee – a professional bodybuilder and eight-time winner of the *Mr. Olympia* title. (1959-)

225. ☺ "One-quarter of what you eat keeps you alive. The other three-quarters keeps your doctor alive."

Hieroglyph found in an ancient Egyptian tomb.

226. "Let food be thy medicine and medicine be thy food."

Hippocrates – a Greek physician who is known as the "Father of Modern Medicine." (460-370 BC)

227. "It's one thing to lose weight, but it's another thing to eat healthy."

Hudson, Jennifer – a Grammy award-winning singer and Academy award-winning actress who became famous during the 2004 season of *American Idol*. She won an Academy Award for Best Supporting Actress in *Dreamgirls* in 2007. (1981-)

228. ☺ "You can't exercise your way out of a bad diet."

Hyman, Mark – a physician, bestselling author and proponent of functional medicine. He serves as chairman of the Institute for Functional Medicine and is the founder and medical director of the UltraWellness Center. His books include: *Food: What the Heck Should I Eat? (2018), Eat Fat, Get Thin (2016), 10-Day Detox Diet (2014),* and *The Blood Sugar Solution (2012).* (1959-)

229. ☺ **"If food is your best friend, it's also your worst enemy."**

Jones, Edward "Grandpa" – a banjo player and country and gospel music singer who was inducted into the Country Music Hall of Fame. (1913-1998)

230. **"People want to think that staying in shape costs a lot of money. They couldn't be more wrong. It doesn't cost anything to walk. And it's probably a lot cheaper to go to the corner store and buy vegetables than take a family out for fast food."**

Joyner, Florence Griffith – "Flo-Jo" was a track and field athlete who set world records in the 100 and 200-meter dashes. She died in 1998 at the age of 38. (1959-1998)

231. **"The body becomes what the foods are, as the spirit becomes what the thoughts are."**

Kemetic Saying

232. **"God, in His infinite wisdom, neglected nothing and if we would eat our food without trying to improve, change or refine it, thereby destroying its life–giving elements, it would meet all requirements of the body."**

Kloss, Jethro – a health food author who is best known for his vegan cookbook *Back to Eden* (1939). (1863-1946)

233. ☺ **"Life expectancy would grow by leaps and bounds if green vegetables smelled as good as bacon."**

Larson, Doug – a newspaper columnist and editor for the *Door County Advocate* (WI) and a daily columnist for the *Green Bay Press-Gazette*. (1926-)

234. ☺ "Food is an important part of a balanced diet."

Lebowitz, Fran – an author and public speaker who is known for her critical social commentary on American life. (1950-)

235. ☺ "Good food is wise medicine."

Levitt, Alison – a physician whose medical practice integrates the wisdom of ancient healing practices with modern medicine. She is the creator of *Doctor in the Kitchen*, which helps people maximize their health and vitality through nutrition.

236. "About eighty percent of the food on shelves of supermarkets today didn't exist 100 years ago."

McCleary, Larry – a neurosurgeon who studied aging brains and became fascinated with Americans' increasing obesity and nutritionally starved brains. His research reveals how sticky fat cells send mixed messages to our brain, which lead to overeating and weight gain.

237. ☺ "It is easier to change a man's religion than to change his diet."

Mead, Margaret – a cultural anthropologist, author, and speaker who rose to popularity during the 1960s and 1970s. Her insights helped popularize anthropology in the West. (1901-1978)

238. ☺ "Anyhow, the hole in the doughnut is at least digestible."

Mencken, H. L. – known as the "Sage of Baltimore," he is considered one of the most influential American writers of the first half of the 20th century and was a respected cultural critic and scholar of American English. (1880-1956)

239.   ☺ "The trouble with eating Italian food is that five or six days later you're hungry again."

> Miller, George – Australian film director, screenwriter, producer, and former medical doctor who is best known for his *Mad Max* movie series. (1945-)

240.   "You don't have to be a chef or even a particularly good cook to experience proper kitchen alchemy: the moment when ingredients combine to form something more delectable than the sum of their parts. Fancy ingredients or recipes not required; simple, made-up things are usually even better."

> Morgenstern, Erin – an artist and the author of the fantasy novel *The Night Circus*. It was published in 2011 and won her the Locus Award for Best First Novel. (1978-)

241.   "BASICS OF DIET AND HEALTH: The basic principles of good diets are so simple that I can summarize them in just ten words: eat less, move more, eat lots of fruits and vegetables. For additional clarification, a five-word modifier helps: go easy on junk foods."

> Nestle, Marion – a widely recognized nutrition expert, professor, and author of numerous articles and books, including *Soda Politics: Taking on Big Soda (and Winning)* (2015). (1936-)

242.   "Unbelievable as it may seem, one-third of all vegetables consumed in the United States come from just three sources: French fries, potato chips, and iceberg lettuce."

Nestle, Marion – a widely recognized nutrition expert, professor, and author of numerous articles and books, including *Soda Politics: Taking on Big Soda (and Winning)* (2015). (1936-)

243. **"Real nutrition comes from soybeans, almonds, rice, and other healthy vegetable sources, not from a cow's udder."**

Newkirk, Ingrid – a British-American animal rights activist and President of People for the Ethical Treatment of Animals, the world's largest animal rights organization. (1949-)

244. ☺ **"We are living in a world today where lemonade is made from artificial flavors and furniture polish is made from real lemons."**

Newman, Alfred – a composer, arranger, and conductor of film music. He became one of the most respected figures in the history of film music, winning nine Academy Awards out of forty-three nominations. (1900-1970)

245. ☺ **"A fruit is a vegetable with looks and money. Plus, if you let fruit rot, it turns into wine, something Brussels sprouts never do."**

O'Rourke, P. J. – an author, political satirist, and journalist who is the H. L. Mencken Research Fellow at the Cato Institute and regularly contributes to major periodicals. He is a frequent guest on National Public Radio (NPR). (1947-)

246. **"We can make a commitment to promote vegetables and fruits and whole grains on every part of every menu. We can make portion sizes smaller and**

emphasize quality over quantity. And we can help create a culture - imagine this - where our kids ask for healthy options instead of resisting them."

Obama, Michelle – a lawyer and First Lady while married to the 44th President of the United States, Barack Obama. The first African-American First Lady is from Chicago and is a graduate of Princeton University and Harvard Law School. (1964-)

247. ☺ "Eating a vegetarian diet, walking (exercising) every day, and meditating is considered radical. Allowing someone to slice your chest open and graft your leg veins in your heart is considered normal and conservative."

Ornish, Dean – a physician, researcher, bestselling author, professor, and founder and president of the nonprofit Preventive Medicine Research Institute. He is well known for his promotion of healthy diets and lifestyle changes to control coronary artery disease and other chronic diseases. Learn more at www.ornish.com. (1953-)

248. "We are all dietetic sinners; only a small percent of what we eat nourishes us; the balance goes to waste and loss of energy."

Osler, William – a Canadian physician. (1849-1919)

249. "Big food companies have their priorities, which include selling cheap, unhealthy foods at high profits."

Polis, Jared – an entrepreneur, philanthropist, and politician. He has served in Congress as a Democrat from Colorado since 2009.

250. ☺ "Don't eat anything your great-great grandmother wouldn't recognize as food."

> Pollan, Michael – a bestselling food author who *Time Magazine* recognized as one of the world's 100 most influential people in 2010. He has written for the *New York Times Magazine* since 1987 and teaches at UC Berkeley where he lectures on food, agriculture, health, and the environment. (1955-)

251. "Eat food. Not too much. Mostly plants."

> Pollan, Michael – a bestselling food author who *Time Magazine* recognized as one of the world's 100 most influential people in 2010. He has written for the *New York Times Magazine* since 1987 and teaches at UC Berkeley where he lectures on food, agriculture, health, and the environment. (1955-)

252. ☺ "The fat you eat is the fat you will wear."

> Powter, Susan – an Australian-born American author, motivational speaker, nutritionist, and personal trainer. She made the phrase "Stop the Insanity!" popular in the 1990s. (1957-)

253. "Sugar is a toxin. It fuels diabetes, obesity, heart disease, and cancer. At the current dose we consume, more than 150 pounds per person every year, sugar and its derivatives kill more people than cocaine, heroin, or any other controlled substance."

> Rath, Tom – a bestselling author and researcher on health and wellbeing. He has served as a senior scientist, consultant, and advisor at the Gallup organization for most

of his career and is best known for his research findings on strengths-based leadership and wellbeing. (1975-)

254. **"Preserve and treat food as you would your body, remembering that in time food will be your body."**

Richardson, Benjamin – a British physician who was a prolific writer on medical history. (1828-1896)

255. **"The only number you need to remember is 3,500, the number of calories it takes to gain or lose one pound of body fat."**

Rinzler, Carol – an activist and civic leader who has authored more than 20 health-related books, including *Nutrition for Dummies* (2016).

256. ☺ **"The biggest seller is cookbooks and the second is diet books - how not to eat what you've just learned how to cook."**

Rooney, Andy – a television personality who is most popular for his 33-years on CBS's *60 Minutes*. (1919-2011)

257. **"The average person is still under the aberrant delusion that food should be somebody else's responsibility until I'm ready to eat it."**

Salatin, Joel – a farmer, lecturer, and author. He calls himself "a Christian libertarian environmentalist capitalist lunatic farmer". His fans call him the most famous farmer in the world and high priest of the pasture. Those who don't like him call him a bio-terrorist and starvation advocate. (1957-)

258. "This magical, marvelous food on our plate, this sustenance we absorb, has a story to tell. It has a journey. It leaves a footprint. It leaves a legacy. To eat with reckless abandon, without conscience, without knowledge; folks, this ain't normal."

Salatin, Joel – a farmer, lecturer, and author. He calls himself "a Christian libertarian environmentalist capitalist lunatic farmer". His fans call him the most famous farmer in the world and high priest of the pasture. Those who don't like him call him a bio-terrorist and starvation advocate. (1957-)

259. ☺ "Life is too short not to eat raw and it's even shorter if you don't."

Sarantakis, Marie – an attorney, author, and former model. Her book *Essentially Raw* is an introduction to the raw food lifestyle. She advises people aim to eat 51% raw and recommends a gradual approach of introducing more fruits and vegetables into one's diet. (1989-)

260. ☺ "My advice if you insist on slimming: Eat as much as you like – just don't swallow it."

Secombe, Harry – a Welsh comedian, singer, BBC radio celebrity, and actor. (1921-2001)

261. "Patience is the secret to good food."

Simmons, Gail – Canadian cookbook author and food writer who has been a judge on the popular television show *Top Chef* since it began in 2006. (1976-)

262. "Pure water is the world's first and foremost medicine."

Slovakian Proverb

263. ☺ "You can do a lot for your diet by eliminating foods that have mascots."

Spiker, Ted – a professor and chair of the Department of Journalism at the University of Florida. He is a bestselling author whose writing is focused on health, fitness, and weight management.

264. "Recipes are important but only to a point. What's more important than recipes is how we think about food, and a good cookbook should open up a new way of doing just that."

Symon, Michael – a chef, restaurateur, television personality, and author. (1969-)

265. ☺ "The most remarkable thing about my mother is that for thirty years she served the family nothing but leftovers. The original meal has never been found."

Trillin, Calvin – a journalist, humorist, food writer, and author. (1935-)

266. ☺ "Water - a thoroughly underrated drink."

Trotman, Wayne – a Trinidad-born British independent filmmaker, writer, photographer, composer, and producer of electronic music. (1964-)

267. "The food you eat can be either the safest and most powerful form of medicine or the slowest form of poison."

Wigmore, Ann – a Lithuanian-American holistic health practitioner, nutritionist, and author. (1909-1993)

268. "No single food will make or break good health. But the kinds of food you choose day in and day out have a major impact."

> Willet, Walter – a physician and one of the world's most influential nutritionists. He is a Harvard professor who has published more than 1,500 scientific articles on diet and disease, and is best known for his 2001 book *Eat, Drink, and Be Healthy*. (1945-)

269. "A diet rich in fruits and vegetables plays a role in reducing the risk of all the major causes of illness and death."

> Willet, Walter – a physician and one of the world's most influential nutritionists. He is a Harvard professor who has published more than 1,500 scientific articles on diet and disease, and is best known for his 2001 book *Eat, Drink, and Be Healthy*. (1945-)

270. "The human body heals itself and nutrition provides the resources to accomplish the task."

> Williams, Roger – a pioneer in Biochemistry and Nutrition who spent his career at the University of Texas at Austin. He played a major role in nutritional research and discovery and wrote about the importance of good nutrition. (1893-1988)

Health Care

271. "America does not have a health-care system. We have a sick-care system... It's a stretch to use the

word 'system' to describe, as this word denotes organization."

Bach, Peter – an epidemiologist who is Director of the Center for Health Policy and Outcomes at Memorial Sloan-Kettering Cancer Center in New York City. His research focuses on healthcare policy related to Medicare, racial disparities in cancer care, and lung cancer. (1964-)

272. ☺ "And I believe that the best buy in public health today must be a combination of regular physical exercise and a healthy diet."

Bishop, Julie – an Australian politician who has served as the Minister for Foreign Affairs since 2013. (1956-)

273. ☺ "Never go to a doctor whose office plants have died."

Bombeck, Erma – a popular humorist and bestselling author who was known for her newspaper column that described suburban home life. It ran from the mid-1960s until the late 1990s. (1927-1996)

274. ☺ "America's health care system is neither healthy, caring, nor a system."

Cronkite, Walter – a broadcast journalist who was best known as anchorman for the *CBS Evening News* for 19 years. (1916-2009)

275. ☺ "Effective health care depends on self-care; this fact is currently heralded as if it were a discovery."

Illich, Ivan – an Austrian philosopher, Roman Catholic priest, and outspoken social critic of contemporary Western culture. (1926-2002)

276. "The doctor has been taught to be interested not in health but in disease. What the public is taught is that health is the cure for disease."

Montagu, Ashley – formerly known as Israel Ehrenberg, he was a British-American anthropologist who is credited with popularizing the study of race and gender and their relation to politics. (1905-1999)

277. "We know a great deal more about the causes of physical disease than we do about the causes of physical health."

Peck, M. Scott – a psychiatrist and bestselling author. He is best known for his first book *The Road Less Traveled*. (1978). (1936-2005)

278. "The patient should be made to understand that he or she must take charge of his own life. Don't take your body to the doctor as if he were a repair shop."

Regestein, Quentin – a psychiatrist focused on sleep, attention, and fatigue disorders. He also serves as an Associate Professor of Psychiatry at Harvard Medical School and an Associate Psychiatrist in the Department of Psychiatry at Brigham and Women's Hospital in Boston. (1938-)

279. ☺ "Surgeons can cut out everything except cause."

Shelton, Herbert – a naturopath, alternative medicine advocate, and author. (1895-1985)

280. "We should resolve now that the health of this nation is a national concern; that financial barriers in the way of attaining health shall be removed; that the

health of all its citizens deserves the help of all the nation."

Truman, Harry – the 33rd President of the United States who took office after the death of Franklin Roosevelt. He is best known for using the atomic bomb against Japan to end WW II, rebuilding Europe, helping to create NATO, intervening in the Korean War, desegregating the military, supporting an independent Israel, and founding the United Nations (1884-1972)

281. ☺ "The art of medicine consists of amusing the patient while nature cures the disease."

Voltaire – a French writer, historian, philosopher, and social critic. (1694-1778)

282. "Imagine a world in which medicine was oriented toward healing rather than disease, where doctors believed in the natural healing capacity of human beings and emphasized prevention above treatment. In such a world, doctors and patients would be partners working toward the same ends."

Weil, Andrew – a physician and bestselling author on holistic health. He played a major role in establishing integrative medicine, which combines alternative medicine, conventional evidence-based medicine, and other practices into a system that addresses holistic human healing. (1942-)

283. ☺ "A doctor gave a man six months to live. The man couldn't pay his bill, so he gave him another six months."

Youngman, Henny – a comedian and violinist who was famous for alternating between one-liners and violin playing. (1906-1998)

Healthy Lifestyle

284. **"70 to 90% of our chronic diseases are caused by lifestyle choices, not genetics."**

Aldana, Steven – a foremost expert on healthy living and worksite wellness. The quote is from his book *Culture Clash - How We Win The Battle for Better Health.* (2013)

285. ☺ **"Coffee is a beverage that puts one to sleep when not drank."**

Allais, Alphonse – a French writer and humorist. (1854-1905)

286. ☺ **"A car is not the only thing that can be recalled by its maker."**

Author Unknown

287. ☺ **"Do something today that your future self will thank you for!"**

Author Unknown

288. ☺ **"If everything is coming your way, you are in the wrong lane!"**

Author Unknown

289. ☺ "It takes 8,460 bolts to assemble an automobile, and only one nut to scatter it all over the road!"

Author Unknown

290. ☺ "Obviously, you can't change your genes, but you can give them a damn good run for their money."

Author Unknown

291. ☺ "In order to change we must be sick and tired of being sick and tired."

Author unknown

292. "It is important to receive essential sun exposure all year long, preferably every day and especially in the morning. Morning light, entering our eyes, regulates our vital circadian rhythms that control appetite, energy, mood, sleep, libido and other body-mind functions."

Ceder, Ken – a health science researcher who focuses on the biological benefits of light. He is currently the executive director of Science of Light, a non-profit organization in Peoria, AZ.

293. "Unfortunately for millions of people, the advent of the computer age has created an indoor lifestyle of 'contemporary cave dwellers' that are unwittingly starving for light! Weight gain, poor sleep, depression and fatigue are some of the serious side effects associated with being out of sync with the natural rhythm and radiant energy of light."

Ceder, Ken – a health science researcher who focuses on the biological benefits of light. He is currently the executive director of Science of Light, a non-profit organization in Peoria, AZ.

294. "If we are creating ourselves all the time, then it is never too late to begin creating the bodies we want instead of the ones we mistakenly assume we are stuck with."

Chopra, Deepak – an internationally renowned Indian-American physician, speaker, and writer. His books and videos have made him a leading figure in the alternative medicine and New Age movements. (1947-)

295. ☺ "When did you ever regret working out and eating healthy? Yeah, that's what I thought."

Google Images: Healthy Snack Quotes

296. "I want to encourage people to make healthy life choices, whether it's training for a half-marathon, or eating more vegetables."

Grannis, Kina – a guitarist and singer-songwriter who won the 2008 *Doritos Crash the Super Bowl* contest and earned a recording contract. She won Best Web-Born Artist at the 2011 MTV Music Awards. (1985-)

297. "When it comes to eating right and exercising, there is no 'I'll start tomorrow.' Tomorrow is disease."

Guillemets, Terri – a quotation anthologist and creator of *The Quote Garden*. (1973-)

298. "The biggest reason most people fail is that they try to fix too much at once – join a gym, get out of debt, floss after meals and have thinner thighs in 30 days."

> Henner, Marilu – an actress and author who is best known for her role in the sitcom *Taxi* from 1978-1983. She has hyperthymesia, which allows her to remember specific details of her daily life since she was a child. (1952-)

299. "It's about having an active lifestyle, staying healthy, and making the right decisions. Life is about balance. Not everybody wants to run a marathon, but we could all start working out and being active, whether you walk to work or take an extra flight of stairs."

> Ohno, Apolo – a former speed skating champion and eight-time medalist in three Winter Olympics between 2002-2010. (1982-)

300. "Lack of activity destroys the good condition of every human being, while movement and methodical physical exercise save it and preserve it."

> Plato – an ancient Greek philosopher who established the foundations of Western philosophy, science, and mathematics. He also had a major influence on Western religion and spirituality. His teacher was Socrates and Aristotle was his most famous student. (427-347 BC)

301. "Sitting is the most underrated health threat of modern times."

> Rath, Tom – a bestselling author and researcher on health and wellbeing. He has served as a senior scientist, consultant, and advisor at the Gallup organization for most

of his career and is best known for his research findings on strengths-based leadership and wellbeing. (1975-)

302. ☺ "Driving like there's no tomorrow could happen."

Safe Driving Slogan

303. ☺ "The problem with drinking and driving is the mourning after."

Safe Driving Slogan

304. "Moderation is the only rule of a healthful life. This means moderation in all things wholesome."

Shelton, Herbert – a naturopath, alternative medicine advocate, and author. (1895-1985)

305. "Sorry, there's no magic bullet. You gotta eat healthy and live healthy to be healthy and look healthy. End of story."

Spurlock, Morgan – a documentary filmmaker, director, and producer who is best known for the documentary film *Super Size Me* (2004), which earned him an Academy Award nomination. (1970-)

306. ☺ "America has got to be the only country in the world where people need energy drinks to sit in front of a computer."

Vanatta, Mike – attributed to Mike Vanatta.

Prevention & Self-care

307. ☺ "I drive way too fast to worry about cholesterol."

Author Unknown

308. "The body is like a piano, and happiness is like music. It is needful to have the instrument in good order."

Beecher, Henry – a minister, social reformer, and popular speaker who is best known for his support of the abolition of slavery, his emphasis on God's love, and his adultery trial in 1875 that ended with the jury unable to reach a verdict. (1813-1887)

309. ☺ "If I'd known I was going to live this long, I'd have taken better care of myself."

Blake, Eubie – a composer, lyricist, and pianist of ragtime, jazz, and popular music. (1883-1983)

310. "Each patient carries his own doctor inside him."

Cousins, Norman – a political journalist and author. (1915-1990)

311. "Prevention is better than cure."

Erasmus, Desiderius – a Dutch Catholic priest and social critic during the Dutch Renaissance. He was the first editor of the *New Testament*. (1466-1536)

312. ☺ "You have a great body. It is an intricate piece of technology and a sophisticated super-computer. It runs on peanuts and even regenerates itself.

Your relationship with your body is one of the most important relationships you'll ever have. And since repairs are expensive and spare parts are hard to come by, it pays to make that relationship good."

Goodier, Steve – an ordained minister and author of several books. He teaches, speaks, and writes about personal development, motivation, and making necessary life changes.

313. ☺ "Genes load the gun, but environment pulls the trigger."

Heber, David – a Professor of Medicine and Public Health at UCLA. His research and writing interests include obesity treatment and nutrition for cancer prevention. He was included in the Thomson Reuters 2014 list of "The World's Most Influential Scientific Minds."

314. "At the surface, many people's goals are to lose weight, tone up, feel better, etc. But superficial goals get superficial results that usually fade. Dig a little deeper, and the 'why' is usually unveiled: to be more confident, to be more happy, to feel sexy again."

Hoebel, Brett – a personal trainer who is best known for his role on the television show *The Biggest Loser*.

315. "You don't have to be a wreck. You don't have to be sick. One's aim in life should be to die in good health. Just like a candle that burns out."

Moreau, Jeanne – a French actress, singer, screenwriter, and director. (1928-2017)

316. ☺ "It looks as if you have been flossing your teeth too much."

No dentist, ever.

317. "Women in particular need to keep an eye on their physical and mental health, because if we're scurrying to and from appointments and errands, we don't have a lot of time to take care of ourselves. We need to do a better job of putting ourselves higher on our own 'to do' list."

Obama, Michelle – a lawyer and First Lady while married to the 44th President of the United States, Barack Obama. The first African-American First Lady is from Chicago and is a graduate of Princeton University and Harvard Law School. (1964-)

318. "We women know how to take care of everybody so well. But the one person we have written out of the equation is us."

Orman, Suzie – an author, television host, and motivational speaker who offers financial advice. (1951-)

319. ☺ "There must be quite a few things that a hot bath won't cure, but I don't know many of them."

Plath, Sylvia – a poet and short story writer. (1932-1963)

320. ☺ "If you love living, you try to take care of the equipment."

Rand, Sally – a burlesque dancer and actress who became famous for her ostrich feather fan dance and balloon bubble dance. (1904-1979)

321. ☺ "Take care of your body. It's the only place you have to live."

> Rohn, Jim – an entrepreneur, author, and motivational speaker. (1930-2009)

322. ☺ "Good health is not something we can buy. However, it can be an extremely valuable savings account."

> Schaef, Anne – an author and speaker who developed *Living in Process*, her own approach to healing the whole person. It is based on the ancient teachings of her Native American ancestors.

Sleep

323. ☺ "People who snore always fall asleep first."

> Author Unknown

324. ☺ "Sleep is a symptom of caffeine deprivation."

> Author Unknown

325. ☺ "People who say they sleep like a baby usually don't have one."

> Burke, Leonce – a former Canadian professional wrestler whose ring names included "Leo Burke" and "Tommy Martin." (1948-)

326. "The best bridge between despair and hope is a good night's sleep."

> Cossman, E. Joseph – a rags to riches entrepreneur who

made millions marketing things like spud guns and ant farms. (1918-2002)

327. **"Sleep is that golden chain that ties health and our bodies together."**

Dekker, Thomas – an English writer and dramatist. (1572-1632)

328. ☺ **"The best cure for insomnia is to get a lot of sleep."**

Fields, W. C. – an actor, comedian, and writer whose entertaining onstage personality was that of a grumpy man who was quick to use his wit and sarcasm to show his displeasure. (1880-1946)

329. ☺ **"To carry care to bed is to sleep with a pack on your back."**

Haliburton, Thomas – a Nova Scotian politician, judge, and author. He was the first international bestselling author from what is now Canada. (1796-1865)

330. ☺ **"I love sleep. My life has the tendency to fall apart when I'm awake, you know?"**

Hemingway, Ernest – he is considered one of America's finest writers and remains admired for both his writing and his risk-taking lifestyle. He earned the Pulitzer Prize in 1952 for his novel *The Old Man and the Sea* and was recognized with the Nobel Prize in Literature in 1954. Three novels, three non-fiction books, and a number of short story collections were published after his death. (1899-1961)

331. ☺ "There is only one thing people like that is good for them; a good night's sleep."

> Howe, Edgar "E. W." – a novelist and newspaper and magazine editor in the late 19th and early 20th centuries who was best known for his magazine *E.W. Howe's Monthly*. (1853-1937)

332. ☺ "A good laugh and a long sleep are the best cures in the doctor's book."

> Irish Proverb

333. ☺ "Without enough sleep, we all become tall two-year-olds."

> Jensen, JoJo – an author and voice-over professional. Her book, *Dirt Farmer Wisdom* (2002), shares the common-sense wisdom of her grandfather who farmed without machinery or irrigation during the Depression of the 1930s.

334. ☺ "There is more refreshment and stimulation in a nap, even of the briefest, than in all the alcohol ever distilled."

> Lucas, Edward – a prolific English writer who spent his entire career writing for the humorous magazine *Punch*. He was best known for his short essays, but he also wrote biographies, poems, novels, and plays. (1868-1938)

335. ☺ "Work eight hours and sleep eight hours and make sure that they are not the same hours."

> Pickens, T. Boone – a billionaire business tycoon who is best known for his success in the oil industry and as a corporate raider. (1928-)

336. ☺ "No wonder Sleeping Beauty looked so good...she took long naps, never got old, and didn't have to do anything but snore to get her Prince Charming."

Reed, Myrtle – a bestselling author, poet, journalist, and philanthropist. She published a series of cookbooks under the penname "Olive Green." (1874-1911)

337. "Tired minds don't plan well. Sleep first, plan later."

Reisch, Walter – an Austrian-born director and screenwriter who wrote the lyrics to many songs that were featured in his films. He was married to dancer and actress Poldi Dur. (1903-1983)

338. ☺ "No day is so bad it can't be fixed with a nap."

Snow, Carrie – a stand-up comedian and comic writer.

339. ☺ "It is a common experience that a problem difficult at night is resolved in the morning after the committee of sleep has worked on it."

Steinbeck, John – one of America's most influential novelists who authored 27 books, including classics of Western literature like *The Red Pony* (1933), *Of Mice and Men* (1937), the Pulitzer Prize-winning *The Grapes of Wrath* (1939), and *The Pearl* (1947). He was awarded the Nobel Prize in Literature in 1962. (1902-1968)

Weight Management

340. ☺ "It is bad to suppress laughter. It goes back down and spreads to your hips."

Allen, Fred – one of the most admired and listened to comedians on the radio. He was often censored for his unacceptable content, but his style and technique had a big influence on comedians who came after him. (1894-1956)

341. ☺ "I keep trying to lose weight... but it keeps finding me!"

Author Unknown

342. ☺ "If you hang your swimsuit, on the refrigerator door, the goodies inside, will be easier to ignore."

Author Unknown

343. ☺ "If your dog is fat, you're not getting enough exercise."

Author Unknown

344. ☺ "Nothing tastes as good as being thin feels."

Author Unknown

345. ☺ "People are so worried about what they eat between Christmas and the New Year, but they really should be worried about what they eat between the New Year and Christmas."

Author Unknown

346. ☺ "The cardiologist's diet: If it tastes good, spit it out."

Author Unknown

347. ☺ "The first thing you lose on a diet is your sense of humor."

Author Unknown

348. ☺ "The older you get, the tougher it is to lose weight, because by then your body and your fat are really good friends."

Author Unknown

349. ☺ "You can't lose weight by talking about it. You have to keep your mouth shut."

Author Unknown

350. ☺ "Dieting is wishful shrinking."

Author Unknown

351. ☺ "I recently had my annual physical examination, which I get once every seven years, and when the nurse weighed me, I was shocked to discover how much stronger the Earth's gravitational pull has become since 1990."

Barry, Dave – a Pulitzer Prize-winning author and nationally syndicated columnist who is known for his humor. (1947-)

352. ☺ "Probably nothing in the world arouses more false hopes than the first four hours of a diet."

Bennett, Dan – a comedian and juggler who has performed on television and applies his physical comedy to business training for corporate clients. He also has a Ph.D. in Mathematics.

353. ☺ "You know it's time to diet when you push away from the table and the table moves."

Cockle Bur, The – a quote from *The Best of the Cockle Bur: A Collection of Wit, Wisdom, Humor and Beauty* (1987), compiled and edited by Harry B. Otis.

354. "The one way to get thin is to re-establish a purpose in life."

Connolly, Cyril – English literary critic, writer, and magazine editor. (1903-1974)

355. "Well, I think probably the main reason people overeat is stress."

Craig, Jenny – a weight loss, weight management, and nutrition company founder. The company started in Melbourne, Australia in 1983 and began operations in the United States in 1985. Today, there are more than 700 weight management centers in Australia, the United States, Canada, and New Zealand. (1932-)

356. ☺ "Remember, you are not a heavy person trying to slim down. You are a trim, healthy person learning how to reemerge."

Cukiekom, Celso – known as "The People's Rabbi," Rabbi Celso comes from a rabbinic family that goes back 700 years. He is the rabbi of Adat Achim Synagogue in Miami Beach, Florida.

357. ☺ "Don't dig your grave with your own knife and fork."

English Proverb

358. "Depriving yourself will, ironically enough, lead to rebelling and weight gain."

Frankel, Bethenny – a television personality, talk show host, author, and entrepreneur. (1970-)

359. ☺ "The second day of a diet is always easier than the first. By the second day, you're off it."

Gleason, Jackie – a comedian and actor who was known for his brash style of comedy, and for portraying the character "Ralph Kramden" in *The Honeymooners* television show. *The Jackie Gleason Show* was a popular variety show that aired from the mid-1950s to 1970. (1916-1987)

360. "When a craving doesn't come from hunger, eating will never satisfy it."

Google Images: Healthy Snack Quotes

361. "There is no lasting glory in rapid weight loss."

Guiliano, Mireille – an international bestselling author of *French Women Don't Get Fat: The Secret of Eating for Pleasure*, and former CEO and President of Clicquot, Inc. The French daily *Le Figaro* recognized her as "an ambassador of France and its art of living." (1946-)

362. ☺ "I go up and down the scale so often that if they ever perform an autopsy on me they'll find me like a strip of bacon – a streak of lean and a streak of fat."

Guinan, Mary "Texas" – she was the first American movie cowgirl and nicknamed "The Queen of the West." She also gained fame as a nightclub owner in New York City during the Prohibition era. (1884-1933)

363. ☺ **"Dieting is the only game where you win when you lose!"**

Lagerfeld, Karl – a German fashion designer, artist, and photographer who is based in Paris. He is the head designer and creative director of the fashion house Chanel and the Italian house Fendi, as well as his own fashion label. (1933-)

364. **"The biggest mistake people make is to try to lose too much weight too fast."**

Oz, Mehmet – a Turkish-American cardiothoracic surgeon, author, and television personality. He is the host of the popular *Dr. Oz Show* that offers health and lifestyle advice. (1960-)

365. ☺ **"In the Middle Ages, they had guillotines, stretch racks, whips and chains. Nowadays, we have a much more effective torture device called the bathroom scale."**

Phillips, Stephen – a popular English poet and dramatist. (1864-1915)

366. ☺ **"Another good reducing exercise consists in placing both hands against the table edge and pushing back."**

Quillen, Robert – a journalist and humorist who wrote about his everyday experiences from his home in Fountain Inn, South Carolina. By 1932, his work had appeared in 400 newspapers around the world. (1887-1948)

367. ☺ "No diet will remove all the fat from your body because the brain is entirely fat. Without a brain, you might look good, but all you could do is run for public office."

> Shaw, George Bernard – an Irish playwright who wrote more than 60 plays and had a major influence on Western culture. He was awarded the Nobel Prize in Literature in 1925. (1856-1950)

368. ☺ "Self-delusion is pulling in your stomach when you step on the scales."

> Sweeney Paul – a Business professor at the University of Dayton and author of a number of books on business.

369. ☺ "I have gained and lost the same ten pounds so many times over and over again my cellulite must have déjà vu."

> Wagner, Jane – a writer, director, and producer who is best known as Lily Tomlin's comedy writer and real-life wife. (1935-)

370. ☺ "My doctor told me to stop having intimate dinners for four. Unless there are three other people."

> Welles, Orson – an actor, director, writer, and producer who worked in theater, radio, and film. He is most famous for his 1938 broadcast *The War of the Worlds*, which created widespread panic among listeners who believed that the fictional news report of a Martian invasion was really happening. (1915-1985)

THE MIND

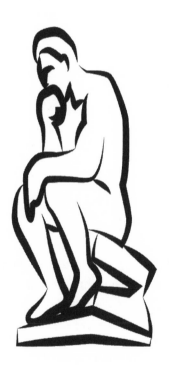

Introduction

"All man's miseries derive from not being able to sit quietly in a room alone." - Blaise Pascal, a French inventor, writer, and Christian philosopher, 1623-1662.

Blaise Pascal said that almost 400 years ago, but what would he have to say about today's "plugged-in" world, where you have to dodge people walking down the sidewalk or across the street because their faces are glued to their smartphones? Can you imagine yourself sitting quietly in a room alone without a phone, computer, television, or music playing? Technology expert Tristan Harris suggests that "we've lost control of our relationship with technology because technology has become better at controlling us." (*The Atlantic*, November 2016)

Increasingly, techno-addiction is afflicting our lives and our minds. The constant stimulation contributes to neural pathways being formed in our brains that lead to addiction - the same process that results in substance addiction. As this process develops, irrational, compulsive behavior robs us of peace of mind and negatively affects the quality of our lives and relationships. Rather than developing our minds through the acquisition of knowledge and seeking meaningful relationships through face to face interactions, we are satisfied with being entertained and communicating through social media. It is going to require a significant effort to reverse this, and it must begin with a focus on our health and wellbeing.

Jon Kabat-Zinn, the person largely responsible for introducing and encouraging mindfulness and the practice of meditation in the United States decades ago, offers a way to unplug from technology and tune-in to ourselves. He teaches that the present moment is all we have. Our lives are lived in moments. Moments are wasted when we dwell on the past or worry about the future – or when we mindlessly fill them with the alluring but empty content filling the screens of our favorite devices. The past is unchangeable, and anything that we want to do to change the future must be done now. So, don't waste the power of now; it's all we have to work with. Rather than living by the popular saying, "Carpe Diem" (seize the day), elevate your awareness to "Carpe Momentum!" (seize the moment!). Strive to be fully present more often in the moments that fill the day - while you walk, listen, eat, work, drive, workout - in everything you do. You have unlimited possibilities right in front of you if you're ready to seize the moment.

Here are my Top 10 Ways for Reducing Distractions of the Mind:

1. Make time for silence each day. Focus on simply breathing in and out and try not to be distracted by your thoughts. Every time a thought enters your mind, return to a focus on your breathing. Start out slowly, maybe five minutes, and gradually increase the amount of time.

2. Take a walk. Walk with a sensory awareness of your surroundings. Enjoy the sights, sounds, and smells that you experience, never letting wandering thoughts take control.

3. Spend time in nature. Unplug from the noise and distractions of everyday life and plug into the beauty and stillness of the natural environment. Smell the roses!

4. Listen to soothing music. Expand your musical taste, if necessary, to find music that relaxes and calms your body and mind.

5. Stretch. Stretching is beneficial for the body and the mind, and for connecting the two. Build short stretch breaks into your day. This is a great technique because it takes little time and can be done almost anywhere

6. Plan the next day, *before* you go to bed each night. On paper or an electronic device, prioritize and schedule all that you want to accomplish. It will help you wake up ready to take on the day, knowing that everything that needs to be done is accounted for, and all that's left is to just do it.

7. Dedicate time each day to self-improvement. What would you like to improve on or learn more about? Read a self-help book, watch a documentary or a YouTube video on something of interest. Spend time thinking about it, and share what you've learned with others. The important thing is to make ongoing learning and continuous improvement a habit that you nurture every day.

8. Clean and organize. Take time to clean up and organize the environments where you live and work. In the culinary world, it's called "mise en place" or "everything in its place," a necessity in an efficiently operating kitchen. Spend a small amount of time each day maintaining cleanliness and order. This frees the mind for other pursuits and provides a sense of wellbeing. It also eliminates the stress of having to deal with big clean-ups and disorganized workspaces.

9. Develop healthy habits. Habits conserve mental energy and help you avoid wrestling with decision making. Habits help you take action without thinking about it. Here's how: 1.) Create a cue to remind you of your desired behavior. 2.) Engage in the routine or desired behavior. 3.) Enjoy the reward of having completed the behavior. 4.) Observe, over time, the craving that develops to repeat the process, indicating that a habit has been deeply formed.

10. Reduce your debt. Most of us have some kind of debt hanging over our heads. Having a plan, and taking action to reduce it, brings peace of mind and a sense of control over your financial future. No matter how small the effort, develop a daily strategy for reducing what you spend to reduce what you owe. Dealing with it head-on and taking concrete steps every day will go a long way towards easing your stress.

The Mind section includes quotes in the following areas:

- Achievement & Success, 371-391
- Attitude & Enthusiasm, 392-409
- Challenges, Change & Choices, 410-453
- Community & Culture, 454-466
- Confidence & Courage, 467-474
- Distractions, 475-481
- Effort & Willpower, 482-517
- Experience, Future & Past, 518-531
- Financial Wellbeing, 532-549
- Focus & Mindfulness, 550-580
- Fun, Humor & Laughter, 581-595

Achievement & Success

371. ☺ "It's never too late to become what you might have been."

Author Unknown

372. "It's not who you are that holds you back, it's who you think you're not."

Author Unknown

373. "I do not try to dance better than anyone else. I only try to dance better than myself."

Baryshnikov, Mikhail – a Russian dancer, choreographer, and actor. He is considered one of the greatest ballet dancers of all time. (1948-)

374. "Your chances of success in any undertaking can always be measured by your belief in yourself."

Collier, Robert – an author of self-help and New Thought metaphysical books in the 20th century. (1885-1950)

375. ☺ "If you think you can do a thing or think you can't do a thing, you're right."

Ford, Henry – an industrialist who founded the Ford Motor Company. His assembly line technique of mass production led to the first automobile that the middle class could afford and revolutionized transportation and industry. (1863-1947)

376. "What the mind of man can conceive and believe, it can achieve."

Hill, Napoleon – the author of the still-popular book *Think and Grow Rich* (1937). He was encouraged by Andrew Carnegie, one of the world's wealthiest and most powerful men at the time, to study successful people and report on their success secrets. (1883-1970)

377. "I've missed more than 9000 shots in my career. I've lost almost 300 games. 26 times, I've been trusted to take the game winning shot and missed. I've failed over and over and over again in my life. And that is why I succeed."

Jordan, Michael – a former professional basketball player who is considered to be the greatest player of all time. He won six NBA Championships while a member of the Chicago Bulls in the 1980s and 1990s and was the league MVP five times. He is currently the principal owner of the Charlotte Hornets NBA team. (1963-)

378. "Don't worry when you are not recognized but strive to be worthy of recognition."

Lincoln, Abraham – a politician and lawyer who became the 16th President of the United States, from 1861 until his assassination in 1865. He led the country during the Civil War, preserved the Union, abolished slavery, and strengthened the federal government. (1809-1865)

379. ☺ **"Success is how high you bounce when you hit bottom."**

Patton, George – a colorful and controversial WW II general whose personality and aggressive actions as a troop commander made him a legendary war hero. The award-winning 1970 film *Patton* made a lasting contribution to his legacy. (1885-1945)

380. **"To follow, without halt, one aim: There's the secret of success."**

Pavlova, Anna – a Russian ballerina of the late 1800s and early 1900s. She was the principal ballerina of the Imperial Russian Ballet and is recognized for creating the role of the Dying Swan and for being the first ballerina to tour the world performing ballet. (1881-1931)

381. **"The dreams I only thought about, the ones I took no action on, well they are still dreams. But the ones that I took action on, they are now a reality."**

Pulsifer, Catherine – a Canadian author of self-help books who teaches that we can positively influence how we live, think, act, and react to life's situations. She writes to help people "grow, develop, succeed, and smile!" (1957-)

382. **"A creative man is motivated by the desire to achieve, not by the desire to beat others."**

Rand, Ayn – a Russian-American novelist and philosopher who is best known for her books *The Fountainhead* (1943) and *Atlas Shrugged* (1957). She developed a philosophical system known as Objectivism, which teaches that reason is the only means for acquiring knowledge and rejects faith and religion. Her political views supported a laissez-faire capitalism that supports individual and property rights.(1905-1982)

383. ☺ "After all, Ginger Rogers did everything that Fred Astaire did. She just did it backwards and in high heels."

Richards, Ann – a prominent Democrat who served as the 45th Governor of Texas from 1991-1995. She was known for her colorful one-liners. (1933-2006)

384. "Winning is great, sure, but if you are really going to do something in life, the secret is learning how to lose."

Rudolph, Wilma – an Olympic champion (1956 and 1960) and world-record-holding sprinter. She was a role model for black and female athletes, and a civil rights and women's rights pioneer. (1940-1994)

385. ☺ "You don't have to be famous. You just have to make your mother and father proud of you."

Streep, Meryl – an actress who has won three Academy Awards and has been nominated more times than any other actor or actress. (1949-)

386. "It is what it is. But, it will be what you make it."

Summitt, Pat – the University of Tennessee women's basketball coach who won eight National Championships and two Olympic gold medals. She retired at age 59 after being diagnosed with Alzheimer's. She ranked #11, and the only woman, on the *Sporting News'* list of "The 50 Greatest Coaches of All Time." (1952-2016)

387. **"It is amazing what you can accomplish if you do not care who gets the credit."**

Truman, Harry – the 33rd President of the United States who took office after the death of Franklin Roosevelt. He is best known for using the atomic bomb against Japan to end WW II, rebuilding Europe, helping to create NATO, intervening in the Korean War, desegregating the military, supporting an independent Israel, and founding the United Nations (1884-1972)

388. ☺ **"All my life, I always wanted to be somebody. Now I see that I should have been more specific."**

Wagner, Jane – a writer, director, and producer who is best known as Lily Tomlin's comedy writer and real-life wife. (1935-)

389. ☺ **"I couldn't wait for success, so I went ahead without it."**

Winters, Jonathan – a stand-up comedian, actor, author, and artist whose career spanned over 60 years. He appeared in hundreds of television shows and films and had comedy records released every decade for over 50 years - receiving 11 nominations for the Grammy Award for Best Comedy Album. (1925-2013)

390. **"Don't measure yourself by what you have accomplished, but by what you should have accomplished with your ability."**

Wooden, John – called the "Wizard of Westwood," he was a legendary basketball coach at UCLA, leading them to ten NCAA national championships in a 12-year period, including a record seven in a row. (1910-2010)

391. "You can have everything in life you want, if you will just help other people get what they want."

> Ziglar, Zig – a popular motivational author and speaker. He was recognized as a master sales trainer for almost 50 years and wrote more than 30 books, including *See You At The Top* (1975), which is still popular today. (1926-2012)

Attitude & Enthusiasm

392. "If you don't like something, change it. If you can't change it, change your attitude."

> Angelou, Maya – an African-American poet, author, and civil rights activist. (1928-2014)

393. ☺ "Wherever you go, no matter what the weather, always bring your own sunshine."

> D'Angelo, Anthony – an educational entrepreneur who founded Collegiate EmPowerment. He has dedicated his life to helping young adults create lives worth living. (1972-)

394. "The best way to predict the future is to create it."

> Drucker, Peter – an Austrian-born American management consultant, educator, and author. He has been called the "Founder of Modern Management." (1909-2005)

395. "If you change the way you look at things, the things you look at change."

> Dyer, Wayne – a philosopher, self-help author, and motivational speaker. His first book *Your Erroneous Zones*

(1976) is one of the bestselling books of all time, with an estimated 35 million copies sold. (1940-2015)

396. ☺ **"What other people think of me is none of my business."**

Dyer, Wayne – a philosopher, self-help author, and motivational speaker. His first book *Your Erroneous Zones* (1976) is one of the bestselling books of all time, with an estimated 35 million copies sold. (1940-2015)

397. **"The most difficult thing is the decision to act, the rest is merely tenacity. The fears are paper tigers. You can do anything you decide to do. You can act to change and control your life; and the procedure, the process is its own reward."**

Earhart, Amelia – an aviation pioneer and author who was the first female aviator to fly solo across the Atlantic Ocean, for which she received the United States Distinguished Flying Cross (a military decoration awarded for heroism or extraordinary achievement). She disappeared on a flight over the Pacific Ocean in 1937. (1897-1937)

398. ☺ **"Genius is one per cent inspiration, ninety-nine per cent perspiration."**

Edison, Thomas – a prolific inventor who held 1,093 patents in his name. He invented electric light and power, sound recording, and motion pictures. He is not only considered the world's greatest inventor but one of the most influential people who ever lived. His advancements benefit people across the world to this day. (1847-1931)

399. **"This is your life. You are responsible for it. You will not live forever. Don't wait."**

Goldberg, Natalie – a New Age author and speaker. She is best known for a series of books which explore writing as a Zen practice. (1948-)

400. **"I have never been especially impressed by the heroics of people convinced that they are about to change the world. I am more awed by ... those who ... struggle to make one small difference after another."**

Goodman, Ellen – a journalist and syndicated columnist who won a Pulitzer Prize in 1980. She is well known for her writing on social change and its impact on life. In 2010, she started The Conversation Project, a group dedicated to the wishes of end-of-life care. (1941-)

401. **"Ability is what you're capable of doing. Motivation determines what you do. Attitude determines how well you do it."**

Holtz, Lou – a former college football coach and analyst who is best known for his quick wit and ability to inspire players. His 1988 Notre Dame national championship team went undefeated at 12–0. (1937-)

402. ☺ **"You must start with a positive attitude or you will surely end without one."**

Latet, Carrie – attributed to Carrie Latet

403. ☺ **"Years wrinkle the skin, but to give up enthusiasm wrinkles the soul."**

MacArthur, Douglas – a famous five-star general who played a key role in the Pacific in World War II. Over his lifetime he received more than 100 military decorations from the United States and other countries, including the Medal of Honor which his father had also received. General MacArthur officially accepted Japan's surrender on September 2, 1945, and then oversaw the occupation and rebuilding of Japan from 1945-1951. (1880-1964)

404. **"A twenty-three-year-long study in Ohio determined that people who saw growing older as something positive lived a whopping seven and a half years longer than those who didn't."**

Moran, Victoria – a writer and inspirational speaker. She is the author of *Younger by the Day: 365 Ways to Rejuvenate Your Body and Revitalize Your Spirit.* (1950-)

405. ☺ **"I think you should be a child for as long as you can. I have been successful for 74 years being able to do that. Don't rush into adulthood, it isn't all that much fun."**

Newhart, Bob – a legendary comedian and actor who has made people laugh with his deadpan and stammering delivery for over 50 years. His 1960 #1 selling album, *The Button-Down Mind of Bob Newhart* remains the 20th bestselling comedy album in history. (1929-)

406. **"There is a real magic in enthusiasm. It spells the difference between mediocrity and accomplishment."**

Peale, Norman Vincent – a minister and author who is most famous for his book *The Power of Positive Thinking* (1952), which remains popular to this day. He served as pastor of Marble Collegiate Church in New York City for 52 years, from 1932-1984. (1898-1993)

407. ☺ "You've gotta dance like there's nobody watching, Love like you'll never be hurt, Sing like there's nobody listening, And live like it's heaven on earth."

Purkey, William – a writer, researcher, and speaker on education and leadership. He has written numerous articles and more than a dozen books. (1929-)

408. ☺ "A healthy attitude is contagious but don't wait to catch it from others. Be a carrier."

Stoppard, Tom – knighted in 1997, this Czech-born British playwright and screenwriter is considered one of the most influential figures in British culture. His writing focuses on themes of human rights, censorship, and political freedom. He has received one Academy Award and four Tony Awards. (1937-)

409. "Life is 10% what happens to you and 90% how you respond to it."

Swindoll, Chuck – Christian pastor, author, and radio preacher. (1934-)

Challenges, Change & Choices

410. "Your life – the way it looks today is a result of your choices...What will you choose today for your tomorrows?"

Allen, Robert - Bestselling financial author and influential investment advisor. (1948-)

411. ☺ "I'm making some changes in my life. If you don't hear anything from me, you are one of them."

Author Unknown

412. ☺ "Very often a change of self is needed more than a change of scene."

Benson, A. C. – an English writer who was the 28th Master of Magdalene College, Cambridge. He wrote the words to the song "Land of Hope and Glory." (1862-1925)

413. ☺ "Life is painful, suffering is optional."

Boorstein, Sylvia – a psychotherapist and author of a number of books on Buddhism and the practice of meditation. She is known for teaching the importance of learning from all of life's experiences - family, work, social and political participation, and formal meditation.

414. "We must learn to let go as easily as we grasp, or we will find our hands full and our minds empty."

Buscaglia, Leo – an author, motivational speaker, and a professor at the University of Southern California. Moved by a student's suicide, he began a non-credit class called "Love 1A," which became his first book titled *LOVE*. His televised lectures were very popular in the 1980s. At one point, five of his books were all *New York Times* best sellers. (1924-1998)

415. "You have to let go of who you were to become who you will be."

Bushnell, Candace – an author and columnist who wrote *Sex in the City*. She followed up her bestseller with six more international bestselling novels: *4 Blondes* (2001), *Trading*

Up (2003), *Lipstick Jungle* (2005), *One Fifth Avenue* (2008), *The Carrie Diaries* (2010), and *Summer and the City* (2011). (1958-)

416. "To get through the hardest journey we need take only one step at a time, but we must keep on stepping."

Chinese Proverb

417. "The self is not something ready-made, but something in continuous formation through choice of action."

Dewey, John – a philosopher, psychologist, and educational reformer whose ideas have influenced education and social reform. (1859-1952)

418. "We must not, in trying to think about how we can make a big difference, ignore the small daily differences we can make which, over time, add up to big differences that we often cannot foresee."

Edelman, Marian Wright – a children's rights activist. (1939-)

419. "Our deeds determine us, as much as we determine our deeds."

Eliot, George – the penname of British writer Mary Ann Evans. She was an English novelist, poet, journalist, and one of the leading writers of the Victorian era. (1819-1880)

420. "All the art of living lies in a fine mingling of letting go and holding on."

Ellis, Havelock – an English physician, writer, intellectual, and social reformer who studied human sexuality. (1859-1939)

421. **"If you don't like something change it; if you can't change it, change the way you think about it."**

Engelbreit, Mary – a graphic artist and children's book illustrator from St. Louis who launched her own magazine, *Mary Engelbreit's Home Companion,* in 1996. (1952-)

422. **"Two roads diverged in a wood, and I – I took the one less traveled by, and that has made all the difference."**

Frost, Robert – one of the most popular and respected American poets of the 20th century. (1874-1963)

423. **"A rose only becomes beautiful and blesses others when it opens up and blooms. Its greatest tragedy is to stay in a tight-closed bud, never fulfilling its potential."**

Galloway, Dale – a teacher, speaker, and author of more than 20 books on spiritual topics.

424. **"Be the change you want to see in the world."**

Gandhi, Mahatma – a political and spiritual figure who led India to independence from British rule through non-violent civil disobedience. Gandhi's approach inspired peaceful movements for civil rights and freedom around the world, including the American civil rights movement of the 1960s. (1869-1948)

425. **"We choose our joys and sorrows long before we experience them."**

Gibran, Kahlil – a Lebanese-born American artist, poet, and writer. He is best known for his inspiring book *The Prophet*

(1923) and ranks as the third best-selling poet of all time, behind Shakespeare and Laozi. (1883-1931)

426. **"The best contribution one can make to humanity is to improve oneself."**

Herbert, Frank – a science fiction writer best known for the novel *Dune* and its five sequels. (1920-1986)

427. ☺ **"Don't tell your problems to people: eighty percent don't care; and the other twenty percent are glad you have them."**

Holtz, Lou – a former college football coach and analyst who is best known for his quick wit and ability to inspire players. His 1988 Notre Dame national championship team went undefeated at 12–0. (1937-)

428. **"In times of great stress or adversity, it's always best to keep busy, to plow your anger and your energy into something positive."**

Iacocca, Lee – an iconic business leader and automobile executive. He is best known for developing the Ford Mustang in the 1960s. In the 1980s he served as CEO of the Chrysler Corporation and his leadership helped to save it from bankruptcy. (1924-)

429. ☺ **"There comes a time when you have to choose between turning the page and closing the book."**

Jameson, Josh – an author of suspense and thriller fiction. He is the author of *A Patriot's Plot*.

430. **"Holding on is believing that there's only a past: letting go is knowing that there's a future."**

Kingma, Daphne – an author, speaker, teacher, and relationship expert who writes on love and relationships.

431. ☺ "We are not retreating - we are advancing in another direction."

MacArthur, Douglas – a famous five-star general who played a key role in the Pacific in World War II. Over his lifetime he received more than 100 military decorations from the United States and other countries, including the Medal of Honor which his father had also received. General MacArthur officially accepted Japan's surrender on September 2, 1945, and then oversaw the occupation and rebuilding of Japan from 1945-1951. (1880-1964)

432. "Don't let your history interfere with your destiny."

Maraboli, Steve – *Inc. Magazine* calls him "the most quoted man alive." He is a motivational speaker, author, and radio show host. His books include: *Definitely Chaotic*, *Unapologetically You*, *Life, the Truth, and Being Free*, and *The Power of One*. (1975-)

433. "Acceptance is the road to all change."

McGill, Bryant – a thinker, author, and social media influencer who focuses on human potential. He is one of the most virally shared and read online authors with over 12 million subscribers across various platforms.

434. "You can suffer the pain of change or suffer remaining the way you are."

Meyer, Joyce – Christian author, speaker, and televangelist from Missouri. (1943-)

435. ☺ "Get comfortable with being uncomfortable!"

Michaels, Jillian – a personal trainer, businesswoman, author, and television personality from Los Angeles. She is best known for her appearances on the television show *The Biggest Loser*. (1974-)

436. "No trumpets sound when the important decisions of our life are made. Destiny is made known silently."

Mille, Agnes de – a dancer and choreographer who was born into a well-connected New York City family of theater professionals. Her father, William C. DeMille, and her uncle, Cecil B. DeMille, were both famous Hollywood directors. (1905-1993)

437. ☺ "Most people would like to be delivered from temptation but would like it to keep in touch."

Orben, Robert – a comedy writer who also worked as a magician and a speechwriter for United States President Gerald Ford. (1927-)

438. ☺ "We cannot change the cards we are dealt, just how we play the hand."

Pausch, Randy – Carnegie Mellon professor who learned in 2007 that he only had months to live. His inspiring September 18, 2007 lecture, titled *The Last Lecture: Really Achieving Your Childhood Dreams*, became a bestselling book and a popular YouTube video. (1960-2008)

439. "I am always doing that which I cannot do, in order that I may learn how to do it."

Picasso, Pablo – Spanish artist who spent most of his life in France. He is regarded as one of the greatest and most influential artists of all time. It is estimated that he created more than 50,000 works of art, including: paintings, sculptures, ceramics, drawings, prints, tapestries, and rugs. (1881-1973)

440. **"Either you decide to stay in the shallow end of the pool or you go out in the ocean."**

Reeve, Christopher – an actor who was famous for his role as Superman. In 1995, he fell from a horse during an equestrian competition and became a quadriplegic. Confined to a wheelchair, he spent the rest of his life as a spokesperson for people with spinal cord injuries. (1952-2004)

441. **"If you do what you've always done, you'll get what you've always gotten."**

Robbins, Tony – a popular self-help author and motivational speaker. His bestselling books include: *Unlimited Power* (1986), *Awaken the Giant Within* (1991), and *Money: Master the Game* (2014). (1960-)

442. **"Nobody can go back and start a new beginning, but anyone can start today and make a new ending."**

Robinson, Maria – an author who earned a B.A. from the Writing Seminars at Johns Hopkins University and did graduate work at the Iowa Writers' Workshop. She is a fiction editor at *r.kv.r.y.*, an online quarterly of poetry and prose.

443. **"You cannot change your destination overnight. You can change your direction."**

Rohn, Jim – an entrepreneur, author, and motivational speaker. (1930-2009)

444. "There are no set limits in life, just those that you place on yourself."

Romiti, Heather – a health and wellness coach and motivational speaker.

445. "It is our choices...that show what we truly are, far more than our abilities."

Rowling, J.K. – a novelist and author of the *Harry Potter* series, one of the most popular book and film series in history. At one point in her life, she was a welfare recipient. Today, she is one of the wealthiest women in the world. (1965-)

446. "The triumph can't be had without the struggle."

Rudolph, Wilma – an Olympic champion (1956 and 1960) and world-record-holding sprinter. She was a role model for black and female athletes, and a pioneer for civil rights and women's rights. (1940-1994)

447. "It's easier to act your way into a new way of thinking, than think your way into a new way of acting."

Sternin, Jerry – a founder of positive deviance, an approach to behavioral and social change. It teaches that sustainable change begins with new behaviors rather than with new knowledge. His career included work with the Peace Corps, Save the Children and Harvard Business School. He died in 2008.

448. "We must always change, renew, rejuvenate ourselves; otherwise we harden."

von Goethe, Johann – German writer, artist, and politician. (1749-1832)

449. "There are two primary choices in life: to accept conditions as they exist or accept the responsibility for changing them."

> Waitley, Denis – a motivational author and speaker who is the bestselling author of the audio series, *The Psychology of Winning* (1979) and books such as *Seeds of Greatness* (1983) and *The Winner's Edge* (1985). (1933-)

450. ☺ "Resilience: The ability to suck it up when everything sucks."

> White, M. J. – a worksite health promotion professional, writer, and speaker. He is the creator of Lean Wellness – an approach to transforming lifestyle behaviors at work through continuous improvement in body, mind, and spirit. (1957-)

451. ☺ "Mondays are the potholes in the road of life."

> Wilson, Tom – an actor, writer, musician, voice-over artist, and comedian. (1959-)

452. ☺ "If you want to make enemies, try to change something."

> Wilson, Woodrow – the 28th President of the United States from 1913-1921. He served as President of Princeton from 1902-1910 and Governor of New Jersey from 1911-1913. After suffering a debilitating stroke in September 1919, his wife and staff handled most of his presidential responsibilities. (1856-1924)

453. "Life turns on little things. The momentous events in history can leave us untouched, while small events may shape our destinies."

Worth, Jennifer – a British nurse, musician, and author who wrote a bestselling trilogy about her work as a midwife in a poverty-stricken area of London in the 1950s. A television series based on her books, *Call the Midwife*, started airing on the BBC in 2012. (1935-2011)

Community & Culture

454. "Volunteering is the ultimate exercise in democracy. You vote in elections once a year, but when you volunteer, you vote every day about the kind of community you want to live in."

Author Unknown

455. "We have to restore power to the family, to the neighborhood, and the community with a non-market principle, a principle of equality, of charity, of let's-take-care-of-one-another. That's the creative challenge."

Brown, Jerry – the Governor of California from 2011-2019 and from 1975-1983. He has served in numerous local and state Democratic party positions in California and was a presidential candidate three different times. (1938-)

456. ☺ "The love of one's country is a splendid thing. But why should love stop at the border?"

Casals, Pablo – a cellist and conductor from the Catalonia region of Spain. He is considered to be one of the greatest cellists of all time. (1876-1973)

457. "We cannot seek achievement for ourselves and forget about progress and prosperity for our community... Our ambitions must be broad enough to include the aspirations and needs of others, for their sakes and for our own."

Chavez, Cesar – a labor leader and civil rights activist who co-founded the National Farm Workers Association in 1962. He dedicated his life to improving the working conditions of farm workers. In 1994, he was awarded the Presidential Medal of Freedom. He was born and died in Arizona. (1927-1993)

458. "The debt that each generation owes to the past, it must pay to the future."

Duniway, Abigail Scott – a women's rights advocate, newspaper editor, and writer. (1834-1915)

459. ☺ "If you put the federal government in charge of the Sahara Desert, in 5 years there'd be a shortage of sand."

Friedman, Milton – one of the most popular and influential economists of the 20th Century. He was an advisor to presidents and world leaders. His theories on monetary policy, taxation, privatization, and deregulation have impacted government policies, including the response to the global financial crisis of 2007-08. (1912-2006)

460. ☺ "Nothing is so permanent as a temporary government program."

Friedman, Milton – one of the most popular and influential economists of the 20th Century. He was an advisor to presidents and world leaders. His theories on monetary policy, taxation, privatization, and deregulation have impacted government policies, including the response to the global financial crisis of 2007-08. (1912-2006)

461. ☺ **"Blessed are the young for they shall inherit the national debt."**

Hoover, Herbert – a politician who served as the 31st President of the United States from 1929-1933. The Great Depression began and lasted throughout his presidency. (1874-1964)

462. **"Ask not what your country can do for you, ask what you can do for your country."**

Kennedy, John F. – "JFK" was a politician from Massachusetts who became the 35th President of the United States, from January 1961 until his assassination in November 1963. Prior to becoming President, he served as a Democratic congressman and senator. (1917-1963)

463. ☺ **"All people are born alike - except Republicans and Democrats."**

Marx, Groucho – a comedian who starred in film and television. He was a master of quick wit and is considered to be one of the best comedians of the modern era. (1890-1977)

464. **"True health care reform cannot happen in Washington. It has to happen in our kitchens, in our homes, in our communities. All health care is personal."**

Oz, Mehmet – a Turkish-American cardiothoracic surgeon, author, and television personality. He is the host of the popular *Dr. Oz Show*, which offers health and lifestyle advice. (1960-)

465. ☺ "It's not the voting that's democracy, it's the counting."

> Stoppard, Tom – knighted in 1997, this Czech-born British playwright and screenwriter is considered one of the most influential figures in British culture. His writing focuses on themes of human rights, censorship, and political freedom. He has received one Academy Award and four Tony Awards. (1937-)

466. "Our culture has accepted two huge lies. The first is that if you disagree with someone's lifestyle, you must fear or hate them. The second is that to love someone means you agree with everything they believe or do. Both are nonsense. You don't have to compromise convictions to be compassionate."

> Warren, Rick – an evangelical Christian pastor and author who is the founder and senior pastor of Saddleback Church in Lake Forest, CA, the 8th largest church in the United States. He is a bestselling author of many Christian books and is best known for *The Purpose Driven Life* (2002). (1954-)

Confidence & Courage

467. "Have the courage to accept what you can't alter and to alter what you can't accept."

> Author Unknown

468. "All that is necessary to break the spell of inertia and frustration is this: Act as if it were impossible to fail."

Brande, Dorothea – a writer and editor whose book *Becoming a Writer* (1934) is still in print. She also wrote *Wake Up and Live* (1936), which sold over two million copies and was made into a musical by Twentieth Century Fox in 1937. (1893-1948)

469. "If you are not afraid of the voices inside you, you will not fear the critics outside you."

Goldberg, Natalie – a New Age author and speaker; she is best known for a series of books which explore writing as a Zen practice. (1948-)

470. "The only courage that matters is the kind that gets you from one moment to the next."

McLaughlin, Mignon – a journalist and author who began publishing aphorisms in the 1950s. He collected them into three books: *The Neurotic's Notebook*, *The Second Neurotic's Notebook*, and *The Complete Neurotic's Notebook*. (1913-1983)

471. ☺ Christopher Robin to Pooh: "Promise me you'll always remember: You're braver than you believe, and stronger than you seem, and smarter than you think."

Milne, A.A. – an English author of books and poems for children who is best known for his books about Winnie-the-Pooh. (1882-1956)

472. "Life shrinks or expands in proportion to one's courage."

Nin, Anais – a French-born American author who wrote journals from the age of 11 to shortly before her death more than 60 years later. Much of her work was published after her death. (1903-1977)

473. "Your silence gives consent."

Plato – an ancient Greek philosopher who established the foundations of Western philosophy, science, and mathematics. He also had a major influence on Western religion and spirituality. His teacher was Socrates and Aristotle was his most famous student. (427-347 BC)

474. "Go confidently in the direction of your dreams. Live the life you have imagined."

Thoreau, Henry – an essayist, poet, philosopher, abolitionist, naturalist, surveyor, and historian. He is best known for his book *Walden*, which was his reflection on living simply in nature. His writings laid the foundation for modern-day environmentalism. (1817-1862)

Distractions

475. "When you fight something, you're tied to it forever. As long as you're fighting it, you're giving it power."

de Mello, Anthony – a Catholic priest from India who also was a psychotherapist, spiritual teacher, and author. He is well known for his storytelling, which incorporated mystical traditions from the East and the West. (1931-1987)

476. "In short, we've lost control of our relationship with technology because technology has become better at controlling us."

Harris, Tristan – called the "closest thing Silicon Valley has to a conscience" by The Atlantic magazine, was the former Design Ethicist at Google. He became a world expert on how technology steers the thoughts, actions, and relationships that structure two billion people's lives, leaving Google to engage public conversation about the issue.

477. **"McDonald's hooks us by appealing to our bodies' craving for certain flavors; Facebook, Instagram, and Twitter hook us by delivering what psychologists call "variable rewards." Messages, photos, and "likes" appear on no set schedule, so we check for them compulsively, never sure when we'll receive that dopamine-activating prize."**

Harris, Tristan – called the "closest thing Silicon Valley has to a conscience" by The Atlantic magazine, was the former Design Ethicist at Google. He became a world expert on how technology steers the thoughts, actions, and relationships that structure two billion people's lives, leaving Google to engage public conversation about the issue.

478. ☺ **"Failures are like skinned knees, painful but superficial."**

Perot, Ross – a businessman and Presidential candidate in 1992 and 1996. He left a position with IBM in 1962 and founded Electronic Data Systems (EDS) in Dallas, Texas. In 1984, General Motors bought control of EDS for $2.4 billion. (1930-)

479. **"Worry does not empty tomorrow of its sorrow; it empties today of its strength."**

Ten Boom, Corrie – the first licensed female watchmaker in the Netherlands. She and her Christian family helped many Jews escape the Nazi Holocaust during WW II, which led to her being sent to a concentration camp. Her life story is told in the famous book and movie *The Hiding Place*. (1892-1983)

480. ☺ **"Muddy water is best cleared by leaving it alone."**

Watts, Alan – a British philosopher, writer, and speaker. He was best known as a promoter of Eastern philosophy for Western audiences. He moved to the United States in 1938 and began Zen training. His book *The Way of Zen* (1957) was one of the first bestselling books on Buddhism. (1915-1973)

481. ☺ **"I can resist everything except temptation."**

Wilde, Oscar – Irish playwright, novelist, essayist, and poet who became one of London's most popular playwrights in the early 1890s. He is well known for witty sayings, his *novel The Picture of Dorian Gray*, his plays, and the circumstances surrounding his imprisonment and early death. (1854-1900)

Effort & Willpower

482. "Water does not resist. Water flows. When you plunge your hand into it, all you feel is a caress. Water is not a solid wall, it will not stop you. But water always goes where it wants to go, and nothing in the end can stand against it. Water is patient. Dripping water wears away a stone. Remember that,

my child. Remember you are half water. If you can't go through an obstacle, go around it. Water does."

Atwood, Margaret – a Canadian novelist, poet, businesswoman, and environmental activist. (1939-)

483. "Suffer the pain of discipline or suffer the pain of regret."

Author Unknown

484. ☺ "Those at the top of the mountain didn't fall there."

Author Unknown

485. ☺ "There are three types of people in this world. Firstly, there are people who make things happen. Then there are people who watch things happen. Lastly, there are people who ask, what happened? Which do you want to be?"

Backley, Steve – an English author and motivational speaker. He is a former athlete and javelin world record holder. (1969-)

486. "Find something you're passionate about and keep tremendously interested in it."

Child, Julia – a popular chef, author, and television personality who introduced French cuisine to the American public with her cookbook *Mastering the Art of French Cooking*. Her television show *The French Chef* debuted in 1963. (1912-2004)

487. "Continuous effort - not strength or intelligence - is the key to unlocking our potential."

Churchill, Winston – a British army officer, politician, and author. He was the Prime Minister of the United Kingdom from 1940-1945 and again from 1951-1955. His strong leadership during WW II, opposing Nazi fascism and air strikes, earned him recognition as one of Great Britain's most admired and influential historical figures. (1874-1965)

488. ☺ "It does not matter how slowly you go as long as you do not stop."

Confucius – a Chinese teacher, politician, and philosopher. (551-479 BC)

489. "A journey of a thousand miles begins with a single step."

Confucius or Lao-Tzu

Confucius – a Chinese teacher, politician, and philosopher. (551-479 BC)

Lao-Tzu – an ancient Chinese philosopher and writer. He is believed to have authored the *Tao Te Ching* and is considered the "Father of Taoism." (Died in 531 BC)

490. "Two little words that can make the difference: START NOW."

Crowley, Mary – a businesswoman who founded Home Interiors & Gifts. (1915-1986)

491. ☺ "If we all did the things we are capable of, we would astound ourselves."

Edison, Thomas – a prolific inventor who held 1,093 patents in his name. He invented electric light and power, sound recording, and motion pictures. He is not only considered the world's greatest inventor but one of the most influential people who ever lived. His advancements benefit people across the world to this day. (1847-1931)

492. ☺ **"The world is moving so fast these days that the one who says it can't be done is generally interrupted by someone doing it."**

Fosdick, Harry – one of the most prominent liberal ministers of the early 20th Century. He served as pastor at New York City's First Presbyterian Church and at the inter-denominational Riverside Church. (1878-1969)

493. **"Start by doing what's necessary; then do what's possible; and suddenly you are doing the impossible."**

Francis of Assisi – an Italian preacher who became one of the most recognized spiritual leaders in history. He taught a way of life that embraced poverty and simplicity. Over the centuries, men and women from around the world joined Franciscan religious orders that imitated Francis's simple way of life. (1182-1226)

494. **"Do not wait; the time will never be 'just right.' Start where you stand, and work with whatever tools you may have at your command, and better tools will be found as you go along."**

Herbert, George – a Welsh-born poet, orator, and Anglican priest. (1593-1633)

495. **"If you want something you've never had, you must be willing to do something you've never done."**

Jefferson, Thomas – a Founding Father, principal author of the Declaration of Independence, and second United

States Vice President (under John Adams). He became the third President of the United States in 1800. (1743-1826)

496. ☺ **"The difference between ordinary and extraordinary is that little extra."**

Johnson, Jimmy – a football broadcaster and former coach who won a National Championship at the University of Miami (1987) and two Super Bowl Championships with the NFL's Dallas Cowboys in 1992 and 1993. He was the first coach to win both a college National Championship and a Super Bowl (Barry Switzer and Pete Carroll have since also done it). (1943-)

497. ☺ **"I am a great believer in luck, and I find that the harder I work the more I have of it."**

Leacock, Stephen – a Canadian teacher, writer, and humorist. He became one of the best-known English-speaking humorists in the world. (1869-1944)

498. ☺ **"I fear not the man who has practiced 10,000 kicks once, but I fear the man who has practiced one kick 10,000 times."**

Lee, Bruce – an American-born Chinese martial artist, philosopher, and filmmaker. He is considered to be one of the most influential martial artists of all time and a pop culture icon of the 20th century. He is also credited with helping to change the way Asians were presented in American films. (1940-1973)

499. ☺ **"You can't wait for inspiration. You have to go after it with a club."**

London, Jack – a novelist, journalist, and social activist. He was one of the first fiction writers to obtain worldwide celebrity status and earned a large fortune from it, His most famous books include *The Call of the Wild* (1903) and *White Fang* (1906). (1876-1916)

500. ☺ **"Don't put off for tomorrow what you can do today because if you enjoy it today, you can do it again tomorrow."**

Michener, James – a bestselling author of more than 40 books. His long works of historical fiction cover many generations in specific geographic locations. His bestsellers *Hawaii*, *Alaska*, *Texas*, and *Poland* are examples of this. (1907-1997)

501. ☺ **"Doing nothing is very hard to do...you never know when you're finished."**

Nielsen, Leslie – a Canadian-American actor and comedian who appeared in more than 100 films and over 150 television programs. (1926-2010)

502. **"At any time, you can rethink your life and reinvent yourself."**

Pitre, Denise – a psychotherapist in psycho kinesiology, where she works with the body and emotional memories to help heal emotional and psychological diseases and illnesses. She coaches people on how to deliberately create or change their destiny.

503. **"You must do the thing you think you cannot do."**

Roosevelt, Eleanor – a politician, diplomat, and activist. She was First Lady during United States President Franklin Roosevelt's term of office from 1933-1945. (1884-1962)

504. "Do what you can, with what you have, where you are."

Roosevelt, Theodore – Mount Rushmore-enshrined 26th President of the United States who served from 1901-1909. He overcame childhood health problems through a strenuous lifestyle that earned him a reputation as a rugged "cowboy." He was also well known for being an author, explorer, naturalist, and soldier. (1858-1919)

505. "Every strike brings me closer to the next home run."

Ruth, Babe – a professional baseball player from 1914-1935. He is one of history's greatest sports heroes and is considered one of the best baseball players of all time. His colorful personality and off-the-field behavior made him a larger-than-life figure in American culture. (1895-1948)

506. "There are no shortcuts to anyplace worth going."

Sills, Beverly – a high-profile operatic soprano who performed from 1945-1980. She was featured on the cover of *Time Magazine* in 1971, where she was described as "America's Queen of Opera." She was also admired for her charitable work for the prevention and treatment of birth defects. (1929-2007)

507. ☺ "You can lead a horse to water, but you can't make him participate in synchronized diving."

Soup, Dr. Cuthbert – born Jerry Swallow, he began his career in Seattle as a stand-up comic before turning his attention to screenwriting and writing books for children under the penname, "Dr. Cuthbert Soup."

508. ☺ "By perseverance the snail reached the ark."

Spurgeon, Charles – a British Baptist preacher who was known as the "Prince of Preachers." (1834-1892)

509. "A spiritual seeker's first duty is to have good control over the tongue. Without control of the tongue we can forget about spirituality. Control in both ways: eating and talking. All the senses are controlled if the tongue is controlled."

Swami Satchidananda – an Indian spiritual teacher and master yogi who was popular for his humorous parables and developed a large following in the West. He was the author of many books and also updated traditional handbooks of yoga. (1914-2002)

510. "He who controls others may be powerful, but he who has mastered himself is mightier still."

Tao Te Ching – a Chinese classic text whose true authorship and date of composition are debated – the oldest excavated text dates back to the late 4th century BC. It influenced Taoism, Confucianism, and Chinese Buddhism.

511. "We should be taught not to wait for inspiration to start a thing. Action always generates inspiration. Inspiration seldom generates action."

Tibolt, Frank – an author and businessman who shares his passion for studying the methods and habits of successful people in his self-help course *A Touch of Greatness*. (1897-1989)

512. **"Little by little, one travels far."**

Tolkien, J.R.R. – an English author, poet, and university professor who is best known for his fantasy trilogy of *The Hobbit*, *The Lord of the Rings*, and *The Silmarillion*. (1892-1973)

513. **"If you hear a voice within you saying, 'You are not a painter,' then by all means paint, and that voice will be silenced."**

Van Gogh, Vincent – a Dutch painter who is one of the most influential artists in history. He created almost 2,100 works of art, most of them during his last two years of life in France, where he committed suicide at age 37. His art focused on landscapes, still life, portraits, and self-portraits. (1853-1890)

514. **"The distance doesn't matter; it's only the first step that is difficult."**

Vichy-Chamrond, Marie Anne de – a French hostess and patron of the arts. (1697-1780)

515. **"I have been impressed with the urgency of doing. Knowing is not enough; we must apply. Being willing is not enough; we must do."**

Vinci, Leonardo da – known as the "Renaissance Man," his interests included invention, painting, sculpting, architecture, science, music, mathematics, engineering, literature, anatomy, geology, astronomy, botany, writing, history, and cartography. The *Mona Lisa* and *The Last Supper* are two of his most famous works of art. (1452-1519)

516. ☺ "If you're coasting, you're either losing momentum or else you're headed downhill."

Welsh, Joan – attributed to Joan Welsh.

517. "Remember, before you can be great, you've got to be good. Before you can be good, you've got to be bad. But before you can even be bad, you've got to try."

Williams, Art – the founder of A.L. Williams & Associates in 1977, which became Primerica Financial Services in 1991. He built a life insurance empire with a simple philosophy: "Buy Term and Invest the Difference" – which sought to get people to switch from conventional whole life insurance to term policies. (1942-)

Experience, Future & Past

518. "My therapist is my journal, which I write in spiral notebooks obtainable for under a dollar in any city in the country. That's why I call my journal 'the 79-cent therapist.'"

Adams, Kathleen – a psychotherapist, author, and speaker who is a leading expert on journaling. Her first book *Journal to the Self* is a classic in the field of journal therapy.

519. ☺ "Journal writing is a voyage to the interior."

Baldwin, Christina – she teaches and lectures through her educational company PeerSpirit. She is an expert on journal writing and has written two classic books on personal writing, including *Life's Companion* and *Journal Writing as a Spiritual Practice*. In addition, she has authored *Calling the Circle*, *Seven Whispers*, and most recently *Storycatcher*. (1946-)

520. ☺ **"The future ain't what it used to be."**

Berra, Yogi – a Hall of Fame baseball catcher who played 19 seasons in Major League Baseball (1946-1965). He was an 18-time All-Star and 10-time World Series champion as a New York Yankee. Berra quit school after the 8th grade but is famously known for his witty sayings. (1925-2015)

521. **"Our history is not our destiny."**

Cohen, Alan – a popular inspirational author, columnist, and radio show host. (1954-)

522. **"We forget all too soon the things we thought we could never forget."**

Didion, Joan – an author who is best known for her novels and essays that explore the disintegration of morals, cultural chaos, and American subcultures. (1934-)

523. **"Don't be too timid and squeamish about your actions. All life is experiment. The more experiments you make the better."**

Emerson, Ralph Waldo – an essayist, lecturer, and poet who led the transcendentalist movement of the mid-19th century, which taught the supremacy of the individual and promoted being self-reliant and independent from societal pressures and norms. He spread his beliefs through dozens of published essays and over 1,500 public lectures across the United States. (1803-1882)

524. "To design the future effectively, you must first let go of your past."

Givens, Charles – a bestselling author of the books *Wealth Without Risk* and *Financial Self Defense*. (1941-1998)

525. "We are just an advanced breed of monkeys on a minor planet of a very average star. But we can understand the Universe. That makes us something very special."

Hawking, Stephen – an English physicist who had a rare form of ALS, commonly known as Lou Gehrig's Disease, which gradually paralyzed him over many decades. He communicated using a single cheek muscle attached to a speech-generating device. His book *A Brief History of Time* was an international bestseller. He served as the Director of Research at the Department of Applied Mathematics and Theoretical Physics at Cambridge. (1942-2018)

526. "Experience is not what happens to a man; it is what a man does with what happens to him."

Huxley, Aldous – an English writer, novelist, and philosopher. He was the author of the literary classic *Brave New World*. (1894-1963)

527. ☺ "That men do not learn very much from the lessons of history is the most important of all the lessons that history has to teach."

Huxley, Aldous – an English writer, novelist, and philosopher. He was the author of the literary classic *Brave New World*. (1894-1963)

528. "My journal is my constant companion. It is never far from my reach...It is a front porch of solace and retreat when I am tired and weary."

> Johnson, Nicole – a motivational author and speaker who is the creator of the "Fresh Brewed Life" philosophy.

529. ☺ "Looking back on things, the view always improves."

> Kelly, Walt – an animator and cartoonist who is best known for the comic strip *Pogo*. He began his animation career in 1936 at Walt Disney Studios, where he worked on films like *Pinocchio*, *Fantasia*, and *Dumbo*. (1913-1973)

530. "Are you doing what you're doing today because you want to do it, or because it's what you were doing yesterday?"

> McGraw, Phil – a psychologist, author, and television host who is one of the best-known mental health professionals in the world. Known for making complicated information easy to understand, his *Dr. Phil* talk show is one of the top-rated programs on daytime television. (1950-)

531. ☺ "A journal is the path of pebbles you leave behind you, so you have the security of knowing you can always return."

> O'Shea, Samara – an author, blogger, and expert on letter writing. She has written two books on the subject and has an online letter-writing service at *LetterLover.net*. (1979-)

Financial Wellbeing

532. ☺ "Before borrowing money from a friend, decide which you need most."

American Proverb

533. ☺ "In God we trust; all others must pay cash."

American Saying

534. ☺ "Christmas is the season when you buy this year's gifts with next year's money."

Author Unknown

535. ☺ "Running into debt isn't so bad. It's running into creditors that hurts."

Author Unknown

536. ☺ "The only man who sticks closer to you in adversity than a friend is a creditor."

Author Unknown

537. ☺ "A nickel ain't worth a dime anymore."

Berra, Yogi – a Hall of Fame baseball catcher who played 19 seasons in Major League Baseball (1946-1965). He was an 18-time All-Star and 10-time World Series champion as a New York Yankee. Berra quit school after the 8th grade but is famously known for his witty sayings. (1925-2015)

538. ☺ "Credit buying is much like being drunk. The buzz happens immediately and gives you a lift... The hangover comes the day after."

Brothers, Joyce – a psychologist, television personality, and columnist. She wrote a daily newspaper advice column from 1960-2013 and a column for *Good Housekeeping* magazine for almost 40 years. The *Washington Post* described her as the "Face of American Psychology." (1927-2013)

539. ☺ "There is nothing wrong with men possessing riches. The wrong comes when riches possess men."

Graham, Billy – a Christian evangelist and Southern Baptist minister who rose to prominence from his large rallies and broadcasted sermons from 1947-2005. He was a spiritual advisor to many United States presidents and was one of the world's most admired and recognized religious leaders. (1918-2018)

540. ☺ "About the time we think we can make ends meet, somebody moves the ends."

Hoover, Herbert – a politician who served as the 31st President of the United States from 1929-1933. The Great Depression began and lasted throughout his presidency. (1874-1964)

541. ☺ "Who recalls when folks got along without something if it cost too much?"

Hubbard, Kin – a cartoonist, humorist, and journalist. (1868-1930)

542. ☺ "Some debts are fun when you are acquiring them, but none are fun when you set about retiring them."

Nash, Ogden – a poet about whom the *New York Times* remarked that his "droll verse with its unconventional rhymes made him the country's best-known producer of humorous poetry." His most notable work was published in 14 volumes between 1931-1972. (1902-1971)

543. ☺ **"The wages of sin are death, but by the time taxes are taken out, it's just sort of a tired feeling."**

Poundstone, Paula – a stand-up comedian, author, and actress. (1959-)

544. ☺ **"Act your wage."**

Ramsey, Dave – a popular radio host and author of numerous *New York Times* bestsellers on personal finance. His radio program, *The Dave Ramsey Show,* is heard on more than 500 radio stations throughout North America. Ramsey's message reflects a Christian perspective on finances. (1960-)

545. ☺ **"Debt is normal. Be weird."**

Ramsey, Dave – a popular radio host and author of numerous *New York Times* bestsellers on personal finance. His radio program, *The Dave Ramsey Show,* is heard on more than 500 radio stations throughout North America. Ramsey's message reflects a Christian perspective on finances. (1960-)

546. ☺ **"People say that money is not the key to happiness, but I always figured if you have enough money, you can have a key made."**

Rivers, Joan – a comedian, actress, writer, producer, and television host. (1933-2014)

547. ☺ "Isn't it a shame that future generations can't be here to see all the wonderful things we're doing with their money?"

Wilson, Harvey – a journalist, gossip columnist, and author who was best known for his nationally syndicated newspaper column *It Happened Last Night*. (1907-1987)

548. ☺ "If you think nobody cares if you're alive, try missing a couple of car payments."

Wilson, Harvey – a journalist, gossip columnist, and author who was best known for his nationally syndicated newspaper column *It Happened Last Night*. (1907-1987)

549. ☺ "Give me the luxuries of life and I will willingly do without the necessities."

Wright, Frank Lloyd – he was considered to be the greatest architect of all time and was also an interior designer, writer, and educator. Over the course of more than 70 years, he designed over 1,000 structures with a focus on harmony with the environment. (1867-1959)

Focus & Mindfulness

550. ☺ "Live everyday as if it were your last because someday you're going to be right."

Ali, Muhammad – a professional boxer who is regarded as the greatest heavyweight fighter in the history of the sport. He evolved from a brash social activist as a young boxer into a person admired for his generosity and for his long battle with Parkinson's disease. By the time of his death, he was one of the world's most beloved and recognized figures. (1942-2016)

551. ☺ "Mental Floss prevents Moral Decay."

Author Unknown

552. "Noticing and appreciating the goodness in a cup of coffee causes us to be happy about living. And the more we notice and appreciate about our lives (and ourselves), the happier we are."

Babauta, Leo – an author and popular blogger on simplicity and minimalism. He is the creator of "Zen Habits," which describes what he has learned while changing habits. (1973-)

553. ☺ "The field of consciousness is tiny. It accepts only one problem at a time."

De Saint-Exupery, Antoine – a French writer and pioneering aviator who is best known as the author of *The Little Prince*. (1900-1944)

554. "Wherever you are, be all there."

Elliot, Jim – a clergyman and missionary who was killed in Ecuador. (1927-1956)

555. "Sometimes the most important thing in a whole day is the rest we take between two deep breaths."

Hillesum, Etty – a Dutch woman and Holocaust victim who wrote about life in Amsterdam under German occupation. She died in the Auschwitz prison camp. (1914-1943)

556. ☺ "No one can drive us crazy unless we give them the keys."

Horton, Douglas – Protestant clergyman and academic leader who was respected for promoting ecumenical relations among major Protestant denominations. (1891-1968)

557. "The greatest weapon against stress is our ability to choose one thought over another."

James, William – a philosopher and psychologist who was one of the leading thinkers of the late 19th century. He is considered to be one of America's most influential philosophers and many consider him to be the "Father of Psychology." (1842-1910)

558. "The best way to navigate through life is to give up all of our controls."

Jampolsky, Gerald – an inspirational speaker and author who is an authority in the fields of psychiatry, health, business, and education. He is the founder of The Center for Attitudinal Healing, which has 130 satellite centers around the world. (1925-)

559. "Everything that irritates us about others can lead us to an understanding of ourselves."

Jung, Carl – a renowned Swiss psychiatrist who founded analytical psychology. His work has influenced many fields of study, including: philosophy, anthropology, archaeology, literature, and religion. (1875-1961)

560. "The little things? The little moments? They aren't little."

Kabat-Zinn, Jon – a leading authority on mindfulness who has made the practice popular in the West. In 1979, he founded the Stress Reduction Clinic at the University of Massachusetts Medical School based on Buddhist teachings. It evolved into a secular and scientific approach that combined meditation and Hatha yoga. The course helps people deal with stress, pain, and illness through "moment-to-moment awareness." Two of his most popular books are *Full Catastrophe Living* ((1990) and *Wherever You Go, There You Are* (1994) (1944-)

561. **"We take care of the future best by taking care of the present now."**

Kabat-Zinn, Jon – a leading authority on mindfulness who has made the practice popular in the West. In 1979, he founded the Stress Reduction Clinic at the University of Massachusetts Medical School based on Buddhist teachings. It evolved into a secular and scientific approach that combined meditation and Hatha yoga. The course helps people deal with stress, pain, and illness through "moment-to-moment awareness." Two of his most popular books are *Full Catastrophe Living* ((1990) and *Wherever You Go, There You Are* (1994) (1944-)

562. **"When we get too caught up in the busyness of the world, we lose connection with one another - and ourselves."**

Kornfield, Jack – one of the key people responsible for introducing Buddhist Mindfulness practice to the West. He is a bestselling author who has taught meditation and trained teachers around the world since 1974. (1945-)

563. ☺ **"Many a time I have wanted to stop talking and find out what I really believed."**

Lippman, Walter – a writer, reporter, and political commentator. He was the first person to use the term "Cold War." (1889-1974)

564. **"What we see depends mainly on what we look for."**

Lubbock, John – a British banker who also made significant contributions to archaeology, ethnography, and several branches of biology. He helped establish archaeology as a scientific discipline. (1834-1913)

565. ☺ **"Don't ever permit the pressure to exceed the pleasure."**

Maddon, Joe – the colorful manager of the 2016 World Series Champion Chicago Cubs baseball team. His witty sayings are known as "Maddonisms." (1954-)

566. **"Your destiny is to fulfill those things upon which you focus most intently. So, choose to keep your focus on that which is truly magnificent, beautiful, uplifting and joyful. Your life is always moving toward something."**

Marston, Ralph – an author and publisher of *The Daily Motivator*. His website has provided a new motivational message every Monday through Saturday since 1996.

567. **"The ability to be in the present moment is a major component of mental wellness."**

Maslow, Abraham – a psychologist best known for creating Maslow's hierarchy of needs in 1943. It describes human motivations as passing through distinct stages based on the following needs: 1. physiological, 2. safety, 3. love and belonging, 4. esteem, and 5. self-actualization. (1908-1970)

568. "Time management is an oxymoron. Time is beyond our control, and the clock keeps ticking regardless of how we lead our lives. Priority management is the answer to maximizing the time we have."

Maxwell, John Calvin – an Australian-born Christian author, speaker, leadership expert, and pastor. He has written many books on leadership, including the bestselling books *The 21 Irrefutable Laws of Leadership* and *The 21 Indispensable Qualities of a Leader.* (1947-)

569. "A mind not to be changed by place or time. The mind is its own place, and in itself can make a heaven of hell, a hell of heaven."

Milton, John – an English poet and civil servant who wrote during a time of religious and political upheaval. He is best known for his classic poem *Paradise Lost,* which was written in 1667. (1608-1674)

570. ☺ "It isn't the things that happen to us, it's the things we think are going to happen to us that drive us almost crazy ..."

Norris, Kathleen Thompson – a popular novelist and newspaper columnist who was one of the most widely read and highest paid female writers in the United States from 1911-1959. She used fiction to encourage values that promoted marriage, motherhood, and service to others. (1880-1966)

571. ☺ "Yesterday is history. Tomorrow is a mystery. And today? Today is a gift. That's why we call it the present."

Olatunji, Babatunde – a Nigerian drummer, educator, social activist, and recording artist. (1927- 2003). A similar version is also attributed to Alice Morse Earle.

572. "Never forget: This very moment, we can change our lives. There never was a moment, and never will be, when we are without the power to alter our destiny."

Pressfield, Steven – a successful author of historical fiction, non-fiction, and screenplays. His struggles to earn a living as a writer, including a period of time when he was homeless and living in his car, are described in his 2002 book *The War of Art*. (1943-)

573. "The most basic and powerful way to connect to another person is to listen. Just listen. Perhaps the most important thing we ever give each other is our attention ... A loving silence often has far more power to heal and to connect than the most well-intentioned words."

Remen, Rachel – a physician and author who has suffered from Crohn's disease for most of her life. She was a pioneer of Holistic and Integrative Medicine. Her curriculum for medical students, called *The Healer's Art*, offers the wisdom of both doctor and patient and is taught in 90 American medical schools. (1938-)

574. "Do you think that I count the days? There is only one day left, always starting over: it is given to us at dawn and taken away from us at dusk."

Sartre, Jean-Paul – a French philosopher, political activist, and author. His work continues to influence sociology and literary studies. He refused the Nobel Prize in Literature in

1964, saying that "a writer should not allow himself to be turned into an institution." (1905-1980)

575. **"An unexamined life is not worth living."**

Socrates – an ancient Greek philosopher and a founder of Western philosophy. (470-399 BC)

576. **"The more you are focused on time – past and future – the more you miss the Now, the most precious thing there is."**

Tolle, Eckhart – a German-born Canadian who is considered one of the world's most spiritually influential people. His books *The Power of Now* (1997) and *A New Earth* (2005) were *New York Times* bestsellers. (1948-)

577. ☺ **"Expect nothing. Live frugally on surprise."**

Walker, Alice – a writer, poet, and activist who wrote the Pulitzer Prize-winning novel *The Color Purple.* (1944-)

578. **"Doing the best at this moment puts you in the best place for the next moment."**

Winfrey, Oprah – one of the richest and most influential women in the world. She is a media mogul, television talk show host, actress, producer, and philanthropist. *The Oprah Winfrey Show* aired from 1986-2011. In 2013, she was awarded the Presidential Medal of Freedom. (1954-)

579. **"I've found a formula for avoiding these exaggerated fears of age; you take care of every day – let the calendar take care of the years."**

Wynn, Ed – an actor and comedian noted for his "Perfect Fool" comedy character, his pioneering radio show of the

1930s, and his later career as a dramatic actor. (1886-1966)

580. "When walking, walk. When eating, eat."

Zen Proverb

Fun, Humor & Laughter

581. ☺ "When people are laughing, they're generally not killing each other."

Alda, Alan – an actor, director, screenwriter, and author. He is widely known for his role as "Captain Hawkeye Pierce" in the television series, *M*A*S*H.*, which aired from 1972-1983. (1936-)

582. "The best clinicians understand that there is an intrinsic physiological intervention brought about by positive emotions such as mirthful laughter, optimism and hope."

Berk, Lee – the world's leading medical doctor and scientist on the healing powers of laughter. He is a professor at Loma Linda University in California where has spent three decades studying how laughter benefits the body and brain.

583. ☺ "Laughter is an instant vacation."

Berle, Milton – a comedian and actor who was the first major American television star. (1908-2002)

584. ☺ "Laughter is the closest distance between two people."

Borge, Victor – a Danish comedian, conductor, and pianist who achieved great popularity on radio and television in the United States and Europe. (1909-2000)

585.   "**There is little success where there is little laughter.**"

Carnegie, Andrew – a Scottish-American industrialist who was a leader in expanding the steel industry in the late 1800s. He became one of the wealthiest persons in the world and gave away almost 90% of his fortune during the last 18 years of his life. His philanthropy especially benefitted social and educational improvements, including over 3,000 libraries that he funded around the world. (1835-1919)

586.   "**A day without laughter is a day wasted.**"

Chaplin, Charlie – an English comic actor, filmmaker, and composer who rose to fame in the silent era of films. (1889-1977)

587.   ☺ "**Laughter is America's most important export.**"

Disney, Walt – a business icon who created Disneyland, Disney World, and The Walt Disney Company. He was a pioneer of the animation industry and introduced many innovations in the production of cartoons. As a film producer, his 22 Oscars out of 59 nominations is the record for most Academy Awards won by an individual. (1901-1966)

588.   ☺ "**Dogs laugh, but they laugh with their tails. What puts man in a higher state of evolution is that he has got his laugh on the right end.**"

Eastman, Max – a writer on literature, philosophy, and society. He was also a prominent political activist. (1883-1969)

589. ☺ "A good time to laugh is any time you can."

Ellerbee, Linda – a journalist who is best known for her work at NBC News. (1944-)

590. ☺ "Start every day off with a smile and get it over with."

Fields, W. C. – an actor, comedian, and writer whose entertaining onstage personality was that of a grumpy man who was quick to use his wit and sarcasm to show his displeasure. (1880-1946)

591. ☺ "Find 100 reasons to laugh. You are bound to feel better, you will cope with problems more effectively and people will enjoy being around you. Besides unhappiness, what do you have to lose?"

Goodier, Steve – an ordained minister and author of several books. He teaches, speaks, and writes about personal development, motivation, and making necessary life changes.

592. ☺ "Laughter is the sun that drives winter from the human face."

Hugo, Victor – a poet, novelist, and dramatist of the Romantic movement. He is considered one of the greatest and most famous French writers. (1802-1885)

593. ☺ "I've always thought that a big laugh is a really loud noise from the soul saying, "Ain't that the truth.""

Jones, Quincy – a record producer, conductor, composer, musician, television and film producer, entertainment company executive, and humanitarian. His career has spanned 60 years in the entertainment industry, where he has received a record 28 Grammy Awards out of 79 nominations. (1933-)

594. ☺ **"You can't deny laughter; when it comes, it plops down in your favorite chair and stays as long as it wants."**

King, Stephen – a widely popular author of horror, supernatural fiction, suspense, science fiction, and fantasy. His 54 novels and 6 non-fiction books have sold more than 350 million copies. (1947-)

595. **"People who laugh actually live longer than those who don't laugh. Few persons realize that health actually varies according to the amount of laughter."**

Walsh, James – a physician, Fordham professor, and author. (1865-1942)

Goals & Motivation

596. **"A goal is a dream with a deadline."**

Hill, Napoleon – the author of the still-popular book *Think and Grow Rich* (1937). He was encouraged by Andrew Carnegie, one of the world's wealthiest and most powerful men at the time, to study successful people and report on their success secrets. (1883-1970)

597. **"It's not the mountain we conquer, but ourselves."**

Hillary, Edmund – a New Zealand explorer who, on May 29, 1953, became the first climber, along with his Sherpa guide, Tenzing Norgay, to reach the summit of Mount Everest, the world's tallest mountain at 29,029 feet. *Time Magazine* named him one of the "100 Most Influential People of the 20th Century." In the years following his historic climb, he devoted most of his time to helping the Sherpa people of Nepal. (1919-2008)

598. "Who looks outside, dreams; who looks inside, awakes."

Jung, Carl – the renowned Swiss psychiatrist who founded analytical psychology. His work has influenced many fields of study, including: philosophy, anthropology, archaeology, literature, and religion. (1875-1961)

599. "Setting a goal is not the main thing. It is deciding how you will go about achieving it and staying with that plan."

Landry, Tom – one of the most successful coaches in National Football League (NFL) history. He was the head coach of the Dallas Cowboys for 29-years. During that time, the Cowboys enjoyed 20 consecutive winning seasons and won two Super Bowls. His 250 career head coaching wins rank him third in NFL history (only Don Shula's 328 wins and George Halas's 318 wins rank higher). (1924-2000)

600. "To tend, unfailingly, unflinchingly, towards a goal, is the secret of success."

Pavlova, Anna – Russian ballerina of the late 1800s and early 1900s. She was the principal ballerina of the Imperial Russian Ballet and is most recognized for the creation of the Dying Swan role. She was the first ballerina to tour the world performing ballet. (1881-1931)

601. "Without goals, you will end up going nowhere, or, you will end up following someone else's map! Develop your map today – set your goals and focus."

Pulsifer, Catherine – a Canadian author of self-help books who teaches that we can positively influence how we live, think, act, and react to life's situations. She writes to help people "grow, develop, succeed and smile!" (1957-)

602. "I started my life with a single absolute: that the world was mine to shape in the image of my highest values and never to be given up to a lesser standard, no matter how long or hard the struggle."

Rand, Ayn – a Russian-American novelist and philosopher who is best known for her books *The Fountainhead* (1943) and *Atlas Shrugged* (1957). She developed a philosophical system known as Objectivism, which teaches that reason is the only means for acquiring knowledge and rejects faith and religion. Her political views supported a laissez-faire capitalism that recognizes individual and property rights. (1905-1982)

603. "So many dreams at first seem impossible. And then they seem improbable. And then, when we summon the will, they soon become inevitable."

Reeve, Christopher – an actor who was famous for his role as Superman. In 1995, he fell from a horse during an equestrian competition and became a quadriplegic. Confined to a wheelchair, he spent the rest of his life as a spokesperson for people with spinal cord injuries. (1952-2004)

604. "Sensible goals or reasons for lifestyle changes - such as 'preventing disease,' 'better health,' or 'weight loss' - sound great, but they exist in some vague future. We burn out long before we actually get there because the promise of a brighter day sometime down the road doesn't make us happy right now."

> Segar, Michelle – she is the author of *No Sweat: How the Simple Science of Motivation Can Bring You a Lifetime of Fitness* (2015) and a sustainable-behavior-change expert who directs the University of Michigan's Sport, Health and Activity Research and Policy Center.

605. "Love what you're doing, and you'll manage to do it - no matter how hard it is."

> Simmons, Gail – a Canadian cookbook author and food writer who has been a judge on the popular television show *Top Chef* since it began in 2006. (1976-)

606. ☺ "People often say that motivation doesn't last. Well, neither does bathing - that's why we recommend it daily."

> Ziglar, Zig – a popular motivational author and speaker. He was recognized as a master sales trainer for almost 50 years and wrote more than 30 books including *See You At The Top* (1975), which is still popular today. (1926-2012)

Leadership & Responsibility

607. ☺ "Deal with the consequences of your actions, 'cause life ain't no video game."

Ikkaku, Takayuki – a Japanese video game developer at Nintendo who has been developing popular games since 2004, including *Splatoon 2* in 2018.

608. "Never tell people how to do things. Tell them what to do and they will surprise you with their ingenuity."

Patton, George – the colorful and controversial WW II general whose personality and aggressive actions as a troop commander made him a legendary war hero. He died shortly after WW II ended from injuries suffered in a collision with an American army truck. The 1970 award-winning film *Patton* made a lasting contribution to Patton's legacy. (1885-1945)

609. "A leader is best when people barely know he exists, when his work is done, his aim fulfilled, they will say: we did it ourselves."

Tzu, Lao – an ancient Chinese philosopher and writer. He is recognized as the author of the *Tao Te Ching* and is considered the "Father of Taoism." (died in 531 BC)

610. "There are two ways of spreading light: to be the candle or the mirror that reflects it."

Wharton, Edith – a novelist and short story writer who was nominated for the Nobel Prize in Literature in 1927, 1928, and 1930. (1862-1937)

Learning, Reading & Wisdom

611. "Reading is to the mind what exercise is to the body."

Addison, Joseph – an English essayist, poet, playwright, and politician. (1672-1719)

612. ☺ "In the case of good books, the point is not to see how many of them you can get through, but rather how many can get through to you."

Adler, Mortimer – a popular author, philosopher, and educator. (1902-2001)

613. ☺ "I went to a bookstore and asked the saleswoman, "Where's the self-help section?" She said if she told me, it would defeat the purpose."

Carlin, George – an influential stand-up comedian who was also an actor, social critic, and author. His subject matter often focused on controversial topics including: politics, psychology, and religion. (1937-2008)

614. ☺ "Books are the quietest and most constant of friends; they are the most accessible and wisest of counselors, and the most patient of teachers."

Eliot, Charles – an academic who served as president of Harvard from 1869-1909, the longest term in the university's history. He is credited with turning Harvard into the preeminent American research university. (1834-1926)

615. "Anyone who stops learning is old, whether at twenty or eighty. Anyone who keeps learning stays young. The greatest thing in life is to keep your mind young."

Ford, Henry – an industrialist who founded the Ford Motor Company. His assembly line technique of mass production led to the first automobile that the middle class could afford and revolutionized transportation and industry. (1863-1947)

616. ☺ "It's called 'reading'. It's how people install new software into their brains."

Glasbergen, Randy – a cartoonist and humorous illustrator who enjoyed three decades of newspaper syndication. (1957-2015)

617. "To teach is to learn twice."

Joubert, Joseph – a French moralist and essayist who is best known for his *Pensées* (Collected Thoughts) which were published after his death. (1754-1824)

618. ☺ "I hesitated before buying a Kindle. I wasn't worried that the digital reader would ruin literature as we know it. Rather, my concern centered on using an electronic device in the bathtub."

Lancaster, Jen – an author of eight memoirs and four novels. After being laid off in 2001, she launched a website and blog, *jennsylvania.com*, to air her frustrations about being unemployed. Her memoir, *The Tao of Martha*, was optioned for a sitcom by FOX. (1967-)

619. ☺ "Always read something that will make you look good if you die in the middle of it."

O'Rourke, P. J. – an author, political satirist, and journalist who is the H. L. Mencken Research Fellow at the Cato Institute and regularly contributes to major periodicals. He is a frequent guest on National Public Radio (NPR). (1947-)

620. ☺ "Two trucks loaded with a thousand copies of Roget's Thesaurus collided as they left a New York publishing house last week, according to the Associated Press. Witnesses were stunned, startled, aghast, taken aback, stupefied, appalled, surprised, shocked and rattled."

Schlein, Alan – a Washington political reporter since 1982 and author of the bestselling *Find It Online: The Complete Guide to Online Research.* He has written the monthly "Washington Watch" for 25 years and runs *DeadlineOnline. com.*

621. "Reading is a means of thinking with another person's mind; it forces you to stretch your own."

Scribner Jr., Charles – one-time head of Charles Scribner's Sons publishing company, he also served as Ernest Hemingway's personal editor and publisher. Hemingway once advised him, "Always do sober what you said you'd do when you were drunk. That will teach you to keep your mouth shut!" (1921-1995)

622. ☺ "Did you know that five out of three people have trouble with fractions."

Trillin, Calvin – a journalist, humorist, food writer, and author. (1935-)

623. ☺ "Wisdom doesn't necessarily come with age. Sometimes age just shows up all by itself."

Wilson, Tom – an actor, writer, musician, voice-over artist, and comedian. (1959-)

624. "My alma mater was books, a good library... I could spend the rest of my life reading, just satisfying my curiosity."

X, Malcolm – an African-American Muslim minister and human rights activist. After becoming a leader in the Nation of Islam and promoting black supremacy and the separation of black and white Americans, he went through a conversion to Sunni Islam and condemned the Nation of Islam's beliefs. He embraced black self-determination and self-defense, and the solidarity of all people of African descent. His life ended when he was assassinated by three members of the Nation of Islam. (1925-1965)

Mind, Speech & Thoughts

625. ☺ "Begin challenging your assumptions. Your assumptions are the windows on the world. Scrub them off every once in a while, or the light won't come in."

Alda, Alan – an actor, director, screenwriter, and author. He is widely known for his role as "Captain Hawkeye Pierce" in the television series, *M*A*S*H.*, which aired from 1972-1983. (1936-)

626. ☺ "No thought lives in your head rent-free."

Allen, Robert – a bestselling financial author and influential investment advisor. (1948-)

627. ☺ "The mind is like tofu. It tastes like whatever you marinate it in."

Boorstein, Sylvia – a psychotherapist and author of a number of books on Buddhism and the practice of meditation. She is known for teaching the importance of learning from all of life's experiences - family, work, social and political participation, and formal meditation.

628. "I insist on a lot of time being spent, almost every day, to just sit and think. That is very uncommon in American business. I read and think. So, I do more reading and thinking, and make less impulse decisions than most people in business. I do it because I like this kind of life."

Buffett, Warren – a businessman and investor who is one of the wealthiest and most influential people in the world. He is CEO of Berkshire Hathaway and well known for his philanthropic efforts. (1930-)

629. ☺ "You can have such an open mind that it is too porous to hold a conviction."

Crane, George – a psychologist, physician, author, and conservative syndicated newspaper columnist for 60 years. He was the father of Republican United States congressmen Phil and Dan Crane. (1901-1995)

630. ☺ "Insanity runs in my family. It practically gallops."

Grant, Cary – a British-American movie actor who is considered one of Hollywood's iconic leading men. (1904-1986)

631. ☺ **"A man's mind stretched by a new idea can never go back to its original dimensions."**

Holmes Sr., Oliver Wendell – a physician, poet, and author who is considered to be one of the best writers of his time. (1809-1894)

632. **"We all talk to ourselves. A major key to success exists in what we say to ourselves, which helps to shape our attitude and mindset."**

Johnson, Darren – an author, trainer, and speaker on organizational development. He is the author of the book series called *Letting Go of Stuff.*

633. **"Our life always expresses the result of our dominant thoughts."**

Kierkegaard, Soren – Danish philosopher, theologian, poet, social critic, and author. (1813-1855)

634. **"Think wrongly, if you please, but in all cases think for yourself."**

Lessing, Doris – British novelist, poet, playwright, biographer, and short story writer. (1919-2013)

635. ☺ **"When all men think alike, no one thinks very much."**

Lippman, Walter – a writer, reporter, and political commentator. He was the first person to use the term "Cold War." (1889-1974)

636. "You can change your world by changing your words... Remember, death and life are in the power of the tongue."

Osteen, Joel – a popular preacher and televangelist who is the pastor of Lakewood Church, a non-denominational charismatic Christian megachurch in Houston, Texas. The Church, housed in a former sports arena, seats 16,800 and averages about 52,000 attendees per week. (1963-)

637. "Change your thoughts, and you change your world."

Peale, Norman Vincent – a minister and author who is most famous for his book *The Power of Positive Thinking* (1952), which remains popular to this day. He served as pastor of Marble Collegiate Church in New York City for 52 years, from 1932-1984. (1898-1993)

638. "It's the mind itself which shapes the body."

Pilates, Joseph – German physical trainer who invented the Pilates method of physical fitness. Pilates increases flexibility, core muscle strength, and stamina while teaching awareness of breath and spine alignment. More than fifty years after his death, his method remains very popular. (1883-1967)

639. "Words have longer life than deeds."

Pindar – an ancient Greek poet from Thebes. (518-438 B.C.)

640. "Discovery is seeing what everybody else has seen and thinking what nobody else has thought."

Szent-Gyorgyi, Albert – Hungarian biochemist who won the 1937 Nobel Prize in Medicine. He is credited with discovering vitamin C and the components and reactions of the citric acid cycle. (1893-1986)

641. "You must begin to think of yourself as becoming the person you want to be."

Viscott, David – a psychiatrist, author, businessman, and media personality. He was a professor of psychiatry at UCLA and one of the first psychiatrists to do a talk radio show that offered psychological counseling to on-air patients. (1938-1996)

642. "We cling to our own point of view, as though everything depended on it. Yet our opinions have no permanence; like autumn and winter, they gradually pass away."

Zhou, Zhuang – known as Zhuangzi, he was an influential Chinese philosopher who lived during an important period of Chinese philosophy - the Hundred Schools of Thought. (370-287 BC)

Productivity & Teamwork

643. ☺ "Don't count the days; make the days count."

Ali, Muhammad – a professional boxer who is regarded as the greatest heavyweight fighter in the history of the sport. He evolved from a brash social activist as a young boxer into a person admired for his generosity and for his long battle with Parkinson's disease. By the time of his death, he was one of the world's most beloved and recognized figures. (1942-2016)

644. "Clutter is anything unfinished, unused, unresolved or disorganized. When you clear your clutter, you create space for new things and your energy and creativity will increase."

Author Unknown

645. "You will never find time for anything. If you want time you must make it."

Buxton, Charles – an English brewer, philanthropist, writer, and member of Parliament. (1823-1871)

646. ☺ "I recommend you to take care of the minutes, for the hours will take care of themselves."

Chesterfield, Lord – a British statesman and a man of letters and wit. (1694-1773)

647. "Things which matter most must never be at the mercy of things which matter least."

Covey, Stephen – a popular educator, bestselling author, and speaker whose message was that people must pursue living principle-centered lives. He is best known for his books, *The Seven Habits of Highly Effective People* (1989), *Principle-Centered Leadership* (1991), and *First Things First* (1994). He was an avid cyclist and died at age 79 from injuries sustained in a cycling accident. (1932-2012)

648. ☺ "The trouble with being punctual is that nobody's there to appreciate it."

Jones, Franklin – a Philadelphia reporter and humorist. His quips and quotes entertained readers of major publications for decades. (1908-1980)

649. "When clients come to me wanting immediate results, I almost always tell them to clear their clutter. Clutter-clearing is modern-day alchemy. It is one of the fastest ways to completely transform your life."

Linn, Denise – a Feng Shui expert and author of 17 books including: *Sacred Space, Soul Coaching*, and her personal memoir *If I Can Forgive, So Can You!* She has been a guest on Oprah, Lifetime, Discovery Channel, BBC TV, NBC, and CBS. (1950-)

650. "Small deeds done are better than great deeds planned."

Marshall, Peter – a Scottish-American preacher who was pastor of the New York Avenue Presbyterian Church in Washington, DC and twice served as Chaplain of the United States Senate. (1902-1949)

651. ☺ "If you can organize your kitchen, you can organize your life."

Parrish, Louis – attributed to Louis Parrish.

652. "Chance favors the prepared mind."

Pasteur, Louis – a French chemist and microbiologist. He was famous for his discoveries related to vaccination and pasteurization. (1822-1895)

653. ☺ "It wasn't raining when Noah built the ark."

Ruff, Howard – a financial adviser and author. His most recent book *How to Prosper During the Coming Bad Years in the 21st Century* was published in 2008. (1930-)

654. "All things are ready, if our mind be so."

> Shakespeare, William – an English poet and playwright who is considered the greatest writer and dramatist in the English language. He wrote approximately 38 plays, among them: *Hamlet, Macbeth, Julius Caesar, The Tempest, Henry IV, King Lear*, and *Romeo and Juliet*. (1564-1616)

655. "Clutter causes stress, and clutter is one of the main barriers of productivity."

> Ward, Charisse – an interventional cardiologist at Tulane University Heart and Vascular Institute. She is board certified in Internal Medicine, Cardiology, Vascular Medicine, and Endovascular Medicine.

Relaxation & Stress Management

656. ☺ "Stress is when you wake up screaming and realize you haven't fallen asleep yet."

> Author Unknown

657. ☺ "Stressed spelled backwards is desserts. Coincidence? I think not!"

> Author Unknown

658. "The truth is that stress doesn't come from your boss, your kids, your spouse, traffic jams, health challenges, or other circumstances. It comes from your thoughts about these circumstances."

Bernstein, Andrew – a professor of philosophy who authored *The Capitalist Manifesto: The Historic, Economic and Philosophic Case for Laissez-Faire.* (1949-)

659. "Tension is who you think you should be. Relaxation is who you are."

Chinese Proverb

660. ☺ "Stress is the trash of modern life - we all generate it but if you don't dispose of it properly, it will pile up and overtake your life."

Guillemets, Terri – a quotation anthologist and creator of *The Quote Garden.* (1973-)

661. "We will be more successful in all our endeavors if we can let go of the habit of running all the time and take little pauses to relax and re-center ourselves. And we'll also have a lot more joy in living."

Hanh, Thich Nhat – a Vietnamese Zen Buddhist monk, teacher, author, poet, and peace activist. (1926-)

662. ☺ "The time to relax is when you don't have time for it."

Harris, Sydney – a Chicago journalist and author of 11 books. His weekday column *Strictly Personal* was syndicated in newspapers throughout the United States and Canada. (1917-1986)

663. ☺ "Worry is interest paid on trouble before it comes due."

Inge, William "Dean" – an English author, Anglican priest, professor of divinity at Cambridge, and Dean of St. Paul's Cathedral, where he became known as "Dean." (1860-1954)

664. ☺ "It is impossible to enjoy idling thoroughly unless one has plenty of work to do."

Jerome, Jerome – an English writer and humorist. (1859-1927)

665. ☺ "If people concentrated on the really important things in life, there'd be a shortage of fishing poles."

Larson, Doug – a newspaper columnist and editor for the *Door County Advocate* (WI) and a daily columnist for the *Green Bay Press-Gazette*. (1926-)

666. "Taking time out each day to relax and renew is essential to living well."

Lasater, Judith Hanson – a yoga teacher, author, and physical therapist who has taught yoga since 1971. She is co-Founder and President of The California Yoga Teachers Association (CYTA) and is one of the founders of *Yoga Journal* magazine.

667. "What worries you, masters you."

Locke, John – an English philosopher and physician who is considered one of the most influential of Enlightenment thinkers. He is known as the "Father of Liberalism." (1632-1704)

668. ☺ "I'm trying to read a book on how to relax, but I keep falling asleep."

Loy, Jim – this quote has been attributed to a few different people with the name of Jim Loy. Jim, if you're reading this, please let us know which Jim Loy you are so that we can give you credit!

669. **"Worry and stress affects the circulation, the heart, the glands, the whole nervous system, and profoundly affects heart action."**

Mayo, Charles W. – a surgeon and son of Mayo Clinic founder, Charles H. Mayo. Some of his accomplishments include: chairing the Mayo Foundation, serving at the United Nations, teaching at the University of Minnesota as a professor of surgery, and serving as a colonel in the Army Medical Corps during WW II. (1898-1968)

670. **"I don't know how to not have fun. I'm dying and I'm having fun, and I'm going to keep having fun every day I've got left."**

Pausch, Randy – Carnegie Mellon professor who learned in 2007 that he only had months to live. His inspiring September 18, 2007 lecture, titled *The Last Lecture: Really Achieving Your Childhood Dreams*, became a bestselling book and a popular YouTube video. (1960-2008)

671. **"Together with a culture of work, there must be a culture of leisure as gratification. To put it another way: people who work must take the time to relax, to be with their families, to enjoy themselves, read, listen to music, play a sport."**

Pope Francis – Argentinian-born Roman Catholic Pope, who is the first non-European Pope since 741. He is admired for his humility, emphasis on God's mercy, concern for the poor, commitment to interfaith dialogue, and his less formal approach to being Pope - including choosing to live in a modest apartment instead of the official papal apartment. (1936-)

672. ☺ "How beautiful it is to do nothing, and then to rest afterward."

Spanish Proverb

673. ☺ "Reality is the leading cause of stress among those in touch with it."

Tomlin, Lily – an actress who began her career as a stand-up comedian. Her breakout role was on *Rowan & Martin's Laugh-In*, which she worked on from 1970-1973. (1939-)

Self-awareness & Time

674. "Knowing what you cannot do is more important than knowing what you can do. In fact, that's good taste."

Ball, Lucille – a comedian and actress who is best known for her starring role in the television series *I Love Lucy*. (1911-1989)

675. ☺ "A person will sometimes devote all his life to the development of one part of his body - the wishbone."

Frost, Robert – one of the most popular and respected American poets of the 20th century. (1874-1963)

676. ☺ "Sometimes we deny being worthy of praise, hoping to generate an argument we would be pleased to lose."

Hightower, Cullen – a quotation and quip writer whose quotations were published as *Cullen Hightower's Wit Kit*. One of his more famous quotes is: "People seldom become famous for what they say until after they are famous for what they've done." However, in Mr. Hightower 's case, he became famous for what he said rather than for what he did. (1923-2008)

677. ☺ "This is a do-it-yourself test for paranoia: you know you've got it when you can't think of anything that's your fault."

Hutchins, Robert – an educational philosopher, dean of Yale Law School and chancellor of the University of Chicago. He was married to novelist Maude Hutchins. (1899-1977)

678. ☺ "There are three types of baseball players: those who make it happen, those who watch it happen, and those who wonder what happens."

Lasorda, Tommy – a former Major League Baseball player and manager who spent six decades with the Brooklyn/Los Angeles Dodgers organization. He was inducted into the National Baseball Hall of Fame as a manager in 1997. (1927-)

679. "Until you value yourself, you won't value your time. Until you value your time, you will not do anything with it."

Peck, M. Scott – a psychiatrist and bestselling author. He is best known for his first book *The Road Less Traveled* (1978). (1936-2005)

680. ☺ **"When a man is wrapped up in himself, he makes a pretty small package."**

Ruskin, John – an English art critic, prominent social thinker, and philanthropist. (1819-1900)

681. **"What you think about yourself is much more important than what others think of you."**

Seneca the Elder – a Roman writer from a wealthy family who lived during the reign of three significant emperors: Augustus, Tiberius, and Caligula. He was the father of the Stoic philosopher Seneca the Younger. (54 BC-39 AD)

Work

682. ☺ **"A company is only as good as the people it keeps."**

Ash, Mary Kay – considered one of the most successful female entrepreneurs in American history, she founded Mary Kay Cosmetics in a Dallas, Texas storefront in 1963. By the time of her death, her company had 800,000 representatives in 37 countries and annual sales over $200 million. (1918-2001)

683. ☺ **"In all my years of counseling those near death, I've yet to hear anyone say they wish they had spent more time at the office."**

Kushner, Harold – a prominent rabbi and popular author. His book *When Bad Things Happen to Good People* was a best seller in 1981. It was written after the death of his son, Aaron, who suffered from the premature aging disease progeria. (1935-)

684. ☺ "I always arrive late at the office, but I make up for it by leaving early."

Lamb, Charles – an English essayist and author. (1775-1834)

685. ☺ "If you love your job, you haven't worked a day in your life."

Lasorda, Tommy – a former Major League Baseball player and manager who spent six decades with the Brooklyn/ Los Angeles Dodgers organization. He was inducted into the National Baseball Hall of Fame as a manager in 1997. (1927-)

Section IV

THE SPIRIT

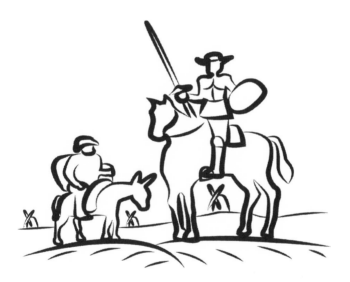

Introduction

"The measure of a life is not its duration, but its donation." – attributed to both Peter Marshall and Corrie Ten Boom.

I have always been bothered by the notion that there's a reason or purpose for everything that happens. Usually, I hear it from well-intentioned people attempting to console someone who is suffering an inexplicable, sad circumstance. In this world, people with evil intentions often find a way to wreak havoc on the lives of innocent, good people, without any apparent purpose behind it. Nevertheless, in everything that happens to us, we do have an opportunity to discover our purpose in it.

First Things First (1996), by Stephen Covey and Rebecca and Roger Merrill, provides a guide to help us discover or create our purpose in life. The authors offer a way to prioritize and balance things in life by focusing on "fully living, loving, learning and leaving a legacy." Here's a simple approach to applying it in your life:

- Live – don't be a spectator; be an active participant in creating the life you want for yourself. Reduce television and phone time; increase time spent having meaningful experiences.
- Love – be grateful for the love you receive and try to multiply it by sharing it with others. Think about who needs your attention and love today; show them that you care. It may be the best thing that happens to them today.
- Learn – continuous learning and improvement should be part of our DNA. Healthy lifestyle behaviors can

change how our genes are expressed. In the same way, continuous efforts to improve can change our lives and lead to desired outcomes.

- Leave a Legacy – sit down and write your personal obituary. How do you want to be remembered? If necessary, start closing the gap between who you are and who you want to be. Make first things first!

Here are my Top 10 Ways to Live, Love, Learn and Leave a Legacy:

1. Volunteer. Volunteering can positively impact your health by making you feel better physically, mentally, and emotionally.
2. Express gratitude. Regularly expressing gratitude has many benefits, including increasing happiness by helping you see things in a more positive light.
3. Reduce stress. Don't get so caught up in the hustle and bustle of life that you forget to take care of your own needs. Nurturing yourself is a necessity, not a luxury.
4. Revitalize often. Find ways to recharge and benefit from increased energy, optimism, and cheerfulness. Go for a walk in nature, call a friend, stretch, journal, play with a pet, listen to music, or find something to laugh about. Discover what gives you energy and get to know when you need to recharge.
5. Live Green. Am I doing more to pollute the world or clean it up? A growing sense of inner wellbeing can increase a sense of responsibility for the world outside. Contributing to a healthier planet both feels good and does good.

6. Wear a smile. Smiling is good for our health and wellbeing. A long list of physical and emotional benefits can be derived from a genuine smile (by the way, genuine smiles are also known as "Duchenne Smiles.") When we smile, we signal to our brain that we are happy. The brain responds by releasing endorphins that produce positive physiological changes. These positive benefits can be shared with everyone around us.

7. Spread kindness. Kindness is contagious, spread it everywhere! Make a conscious effort to extend kindness to others, whether in a random act or something you've planned. Either way, there are real physical and emotional benefits to take advantage of when you are kind to others. When we perform a kind act, our body rewards us with a rush of endorphins that create a feeling of happiness. Recipients of kindness experience the same happiness. And, it doesn't stop there. Even observers of the kindness experience similar benefits! Just one act of kindness can impact everyone around you.

8. Laugh out loud. Research suggests that humor can benefit us in many ways, including: coping with pain, improving the immune system, and reducing stress.

9. Meditate, Pray or Reflect. I am not recommending any particular way to meditate, pray, or reflect. It is a personal and private matter. You are encouraged to do or explore what is most comfortable for you. Making time for this practice will lead to many benefits. It will help you prioritize what's most important, increase your happiness, and improve your resilience.

10. Find inspiration. Inspiration should not be left to chance or random experience. It can be planned for and used to enhance the quality of daily life. Pursue it with a passion!

The Spirit section includes quotes in the following areas:

Beauty, Creativity & Individuality

686.   **"Live out of your imagination, not your history."**

Covey, Stephen – a popular educator, bestselling author, and speaker whose message was that people must pursue living principle-centered lives. He is best known for his books *The Seven Habits of Highly Effective People* (1989), *Principle-Centered Leadership* (1991), and *First Things First* (1994). He was an avid cyclist and died at age 79 from injuries sustained in a cycling accident. (1932-2012)

687. **"Some people look for a beautiful place, others make a place beautiful."**

Khan, Hazrat Inayat – he founded of the Sufi Order in the West in 1914 and taught Universal Sufism. His written works combined his passion for music with Sufi ideologies and led to his claim that music was the "harmonious thread of the Universe." (1882-1927)

688. **"Have nothing in your house that you do not know to be useful or believe to be beautiful."**

Morris, William – an English textile designer, poet, novelist, and socialist activist. He was involved with the British Arts and Crafts Movement and helped to establish the modern fantasy genre in literature. (1834-1896)

689. ☺ **"Be who you are and say what you feel because those who mind don't matter and those who matter don't mind."**

Seuss, Dr. – Theodor Seuss Geisel, who is better known as Dr. Seuss, was a German-American author, political cartoonist, poet, animator, and artist. He is best known for authoring more than 60 children's books that had sold over 600 million copies by the time of his death. (1904-1991)

Belief & Convictions

690. "We all have our own life to pursue, our own kind of dream to be weaving, and we all have the power to make wishes come true, as long as we keep believing."

   Alcott, Louisa May – a novelist and poet who is best known as the author of *Little Women*. (1832-1888)

691. "Prayer is the spirit speaking truth to Truth."

   Bailey, Phillip – an English poet who is known for his one voluminous poem *Festus*, which was first published in 1839. (1816-1902)

692. "With the power of conviction, there is no sacrifice."

   Benatar, Pat – a singer, songwriter, and winner of four Grammy Awards. (1953-)

693. "I try to avoid looking forward or backward and try to keep looking upward."

   Bronte, Charlotte – an English novelist and poet whose most famous work was the literary classic *Jane Eyre*. (1816-1855)

694. ☺ "Faith moves mountains, but you have to keep pushing while you are praying."

   Cooley, Mason – a professor of French, Speech, and World Literature at the College of Staten Island who was known for his witty sayings. (1927-2002)

695. ☺ "One and God make a majority."

Douglass, Frederick – one of the most influential African-Americans of the 19th Century. He was known as a convincing speaker and writer who was devoted to ending slavery and winning equal rights for African-Americans. (1818-1895)

696. "There are two ways to live your life. One as though nothing is a miracle, the other as though everything is a miracle."

Einstein, Albert – a German-born physicist who developed the general theory of relativity and had a major influence on the philosophy of science. His intellectual ability has made the word "Einstein" synonymous with "genius." (1879-1955)

697. "Remember that when you leave this earth, you can take with you nothing that you have received – only what you have given: a full heart, enriched by honest service, love, sacrifice and courage."

Francis of Assisi – an Italian preacher who became one of the most recognized spiritual leaders in history. He taught a way of life that embraced poverty and simplicity. Over the centuries, men and women from around the world joined Franciscan religious orders that imitated Francis's simple way of life. (1182-1226)

698. "The most eloquent prayer is the prayer through hands that heal and bless."

Graham, Billy – a Christian evangelist and Southern Baptist minister who rose to prominence from his large rallies and broadcasted sermons from 1947-2005. He was a spiritual advisor to many United States presidents and was one of the world's most admired and recognized religious leaders. (1918-)

699. "God does not die on the day when we cease to believe in a personal deity, but we die on the day when our lives cease to be illumined by the steady radiance, renewed daily, of a wonder, the source of which is beyond all reason."

Hammarskjold, Dag – a Swedish diplomat, economist, and author. He was the second secretary-general of the United Nations, from 1953 until his death in a 1961 plane crash. In recognition of his leadership and many accomplishments, President John F. Kennedy called him "the greatest statesman of our century." (1905-1961)

700. "For those who believe, no proof is necessary. For those who disbelieve, no amount of proof is sufficient."

Ignatius of Loyola – a Spanish priest, theologian, and founder of the Society of Jesus religious order, commonly known as the Jesuits. Their ministry is focused on education in schools, colleges, universities, seminaries, and on research-based pursuits. (1491-1556)

701. "The hands that help are holier than the lips that pray."

Ingersoll, Robert – a lawyer, Civil War veteran, and political leader. He was made famous for his defense of agnosticism (claiming neither faith nor disbelief in God), which earned him the nickname "The Great Agnostic." (1833-1899)

702. "Faith and prayer are the vitamins of the soul; man cannot live in health without them."

son, Mahalia – a gospel singer who was called "The ~~~een of Gospel." She was also known for her work as a civil rights activist. (1911-1972)

703. ☺ **"God is not dead – He is merely unemployed."**

Kelly, Walt – an animator and cartoonist who is best known for the comic strip *Pogo*. He began his animation career in 1936 at Walt Disney Studios, where he worked on films like *Pinocchio*, *Fantasia*, and *Dumbo*. (1913-1973)

704. **"Prayer does not change God, but it changes him who prays."**

Kierkegaard, Soren – a Danish philosopher, theologian, poet, social critic, and author. (1813-1855)

705. ☺ **"Buddha left a road map, Jesus left a road map, Krishna left a road map, Rand McNally left a road map. But you still have to travel the road yourself."**

Levine, Stephen – a poet, author, and spiritual teacher who is best known for his work on death and dying, as well as making the teachings of Theravada Buddhism more popular in the West. His works often referenced a creator, which differentiated his teaching from other contemporary Buddhist writers. (1937-2016)

706. **"You don't have a soul. You are a Soul. You have a body."**

Lewis, C. S. – an Irish-born novelist and lay theologian who is well known for his fictional works like *The Screwtape Letters* and *The Chronicles of Narnia*, and for his non-fiction books including *Mere Christianity* and *Miracles*. (1898-1963)

707. ☺ "You only live once, but if you work it right, once is enough."

Lewis, Joe – a comedian and singer. (1902-1971)

708. "I have held many things in my hands, and I have lost them all; but whatever I have placed in God's hands, that I still possess."

Luther, Martin – a German priest and theologian who led the Protestant Reformation, which rejected many of the teachings and practices of the Roman Catholic Church. (1483-1546)

709. "In everything, do to others what you would have them do to you."

Matthew 7:12 – from the Bible's *New Testament*, Gospel of Matthew, Chapter 7, Verse 12. The message of this verse is known as the "Golden Rule."

710. "A life is either all spiritual or not spiritual at all. No man can serve two masters. Your life is shaped by the end you live for. You are made in the image of what you desire."

Merton, Thomas – a Catholic writer, social activist, and Trappist monk at the Abbey of Gethsemane in Kentucky, where he lived for 27 years. He is considered the most influential American Catholic author of the 20th century and was a strong supporter of the nonviolent civil rights and peace movements. In later life, he became very interested in Asian religions. The Dalai Lama said that Merton had a more profound understanding of Buddhism than any other Christian he had known. (1915-1968)

711. "Spirituality is seeded, germinates, sprouts and blossoms in the mundane. It is to be found and nurtured in the smallest of daily activities."

> Moore, Thomas – a psychotherapist, former monk, and author of popular spiritual books including *Care of the Soul* (1992). He writes and lectures on archetypal psychology, mythology, and imagination. (1940-)

712. "Religious beliefs and activities can have a profound impact on our mental and physical wellbeing by reducing stress, improving resistance to diseases, enhancing memory and mental function, and helping us to lead longer lives."

> Newberg, Andrew – the founder of Neuroethology – the study of the relationship between spiritual phenomena and the brain. He is a neuroscientist whose research includes taking brain scans of people in prayer, meditation, rituals, and trance states in order to better understand spiritual practices and beliefs. (1966-)

713. ☺ "Practical prayer is harder on the soles of your shoes than on the knees of your trousers."

> O'Malley, Austin – an ophthalmologist and professor of English literature at the University of Notre Dame who authored a book of aphorisms. (1858-1932)

714. ☺ "I would never die for my beliefs because I might be wrong."

> Russell, Bertrand – a British philosopher, writer, social critic, and political activist. He received the Nobel Prize in Literature in 1950 for his "humanitarian ideals and freedom of thought." (1872-1970)

715. **"Heaven never helps the man who will not act."**

Sophocles – an ancient Greek playwright and one of three ancient Greek tragedians whose plays have survived. (496-406 BC)

716. **"For prayer is nothing else than being on terms of friendship with God."**

Teresa of Avila – a Spanish nun and author who is recognized as a Roman Catholic saint. Her writings on prayer remain popular to this day. (1515-1582)

717. **"You are here to enable the divine purpose of the universe to unfold. That is how important you are!"**

Tolle, Eckhart – a German-born Canadian who is considered to be one of the world's most spiritually influential people. His books *The Power of Now* (1997) and *A New Earth* (2005) were *New York Times* bestsellers. (1948-)

718. ☺ **"We may be surprised at the people we find in heaven. God has a soft spot for sinners. His standards are quite low."**

Tutu, Desmond – a South African social rights activist and retired Anglican bishop who became famous during the 1980s as an opponent of apartheid and the first black Archbishop of Cape Town. He was awarded the Nobel Peace Prize in 1984 and the Presidential Medal of Freedom in 2009. (1931-)

719. **"You have to grow from the inside out. None can teach you, none can make you spiritual. There is no other teacher but your own soul."**

Vivekananda, Swami – an Indian Hindu monk who was influential in introducing the Indian philosophies of Vedanta and Yoga to the Western world. He is credited with bringing Hinduism to the status of a major world religion in the late 1800s and was a leader in promoting nationalism in colonial India. (1863-1902)

720. **"I will permit no man to narrow and degrade my soul by making me hate him."**

Washington, Booker T. – an African-American leader, educator, and author who came from the last generation of black leaders born into slavery. From 1890-1915, he was a prominent leader in the African-American community. His autobiography *Up From Slavery* (1901) became a bestseller. (1856-1915)

721. **"There are victories of the soul and spirit. Sometimes, even if you lose, you win."**

Wiesel, Elie – a Romanian-born, Jewish-American professor and political activist. He was a Holocaust survivor and the author of 57 books. In 1986, he was awarded the Nobel Peace Prize. (1928-2016)

Character, Courtesy & Goodness

722. **"The good we secure for ourselves is precarious and uncertain until it is secured for all of us and incorporated into our common life."**

Addams, Jane – known as the "Mother of Social Work," she was an activist who promoted women's right to vote and world peace. She founded Hull House in Chicago in 1889, which became a laboratory for social change. In 1931, she became the first American woman to receive the Nobel Peace Prize. (1860-1935)

723. **"Forget injuries, never forget kindnesses."**

Aesop – an ancient Greek story teller. (620-564 BC)

724. **"What is the essence of life? To serve others and to do good."**

Aristotle – an ancient Greek philosopher who is considered to be the first genuine scientist in history. (384-322 BC)

725. **"A tree is known by its fruit; a man by his deeds. A good deed is never lost; he who sows courtesy reaps friendship, and he who plants kindness gathers love."**

Basil of Caesarea - also called Saint Basil the Great, he was the bishop of Caesarea (an area in modern-day Turkey) and a respected theologian in the early Christian church. He is still widely venerated within contemporary Eastern Orthodox Christianity. (329-379)

726. ☺ **"Treat everyone with politeness and kindness, not because they are nice, but because you are."**

Bennett, Roy – a thought leader who shares positive thoughts and creative insight in his writings. He is the author of *The Light in the Heart*.

727. ☺ **"I nod to a passing stranger, and the stranger nods back, and two human beings go off, feeling a little less anonymous."**

Brault, Robert – a freelance writer who has contributed to magazines and newspapers for over 40 years.

728. "All that is necessary for the triumph of evil is for good men to do nothing."

> Burke, Edmund – an Irish-British author and political figure. (1729-1797)

729. "Too often we underestimate the power of a touch, a smile, a kind word, a listening ear, an honest compliment, or the smallest act of caring, all of which have the potential to turn a life around."

> Buscaglia, Leo – an author, motivational speaker, and a professor at the University of Southern California. Moved by a student's suicide, he began a non-credit class called "Love 1A," which became his first book titled *LOVE*. His televised lectures were very popular in the 1980s. At one point, five of his books were all *New York Times* best sellers. (1924-1998)

730. ☺ "Some people, no matter how old they get, never lose their beauty - they merely move it from their faces into their hearts."

> Buxbaum, Martin – a poet and author whose works include: *Rivers of Thought*, *Whispers in the Wind* and *The Underside of Heaven*. (1912 -1991)

731. "You have it easily in your power to increase the sum total of this world's happiness now. How? By giving a few words of sincere appreciation to someone who is lonely or discouraged. Perhaps you will forget tomorrow the kind words you say today, but the recipient may cherish them over a lifetime."

Carnegie, Dale – a writer and lecturer who developed popular courses on self-improvement. His book *How to Win Friends and Influence People* was published in 1936. It has sold over 30 million copies and is still popular today. (1888-1955)

732. ☺ "Courtesy is a small act, but it packs a mighty wallop."

Carroll, Lewis – an English writer who was known for his wordplay, logic, and fantasy. His most famous work is *Alice's Adventures in Wonderland*. (1832-1898)

733. ☺ "Be kind whenever possible. It is always possible."

Dalai Lama – the 14th Dalai Lama who functions as the spiritual leader of Tibet. He describes himself as a simple Buddhist monk. Born to a farming family in northeastern Tibet, he was recognized as the reincarnation of the 13th Dalai Lama at the age of two. (1935-)

734. "The good man is the man who, no matter how morally unworthy he has been, is moving to become better."

Dewey, John – a philosopher, psychologist, and educational reformer whose ideas have influenced education and social reform. (1859-1952)

735. "If I can stop one heart from breaking, I shall not live in vain. If I can ease one life the aching, or cool one pain, or help one fainting robin unto his nest again, I shall not live in vain."

Dickinson, Emily – a prolific and influential poet who led a very private life in Amherst, MA. Most of her writings were published after her death. (1830-1886)

736. "Character – the willingness to accept responsibility for one's own life – is the source from which self-respect springs."

> Didion, Joan – an author who is best known for her novels and essays that explore the disintegration of morals, cultural chaos, and American subcultures. (1934-)

737. "How lovely to think that no one need wait a moment. We can start now, start slowly, changing the world. How lovely that everyone, great and small, can make a contribution toward introducing justice straightaway. And you can always, always give something, even if it is only kindness!"

> Frank, Anne – a young Jewish girl who became a victim of the Holocaust. She wrote about her experiences in her diary, which was made into the book, *The Diary of a Young Girl*, (or *The Diary of Anne Frank*), which became popular throughout the world. (1929-1945)

738. ☺ "So you're a little weird? Work it! A little different? OWN it! Better to be a nerd than one of the herd!"

> Hale, Mandy – *New York Times* bestselling author and speaker who is known around the world as "The Single Woman." She seeks to inspire single women to live their best lives and to never settle for less.

739. "Help your sister's boat across the water, and yours too will reach the other side." Kindness can become its own motive. We are made kind by being kind."

Hoffer, Eric – an author and moral and social philosopher. He was the author of ten books and a recipient of the Presidential Medal of Freedom in 1983. (1902-1983)

740. ☺ **"The proper time to influence the character of a child is about a hundred years before he is born."**

Inge, William "Dean" – English author, Anglican priest, professor of divinity at Cambridge, and Dean of St. Paul's Cathedral, where he became known as "Dean." (1860-1954)

741. ☺ **"The only time you should look down at someone, is when you are helping them up."**

Jackson, Jesse – an African-American civil rights leader, Baptist minister, and politician who ran for president in 1984 and 1988. He founded Operation PUSH (People United to Save Humanity) and the National Rainbow Coalition to promote social justice, civil rights, and political activism. Rainbow/PUSH is a merger of the two organizations. (1941-)

742. ☺ **"Honest criticism is hard to take, particularly from a relative, a friend, an acquaintance or a stranger."**

Jones, Franklin – Philadelphia reporter and humorist. His quips and quotes entertained readers of major publications for decades. (1908-1980)

743. **"The ultimate measure of a man is not where he stands in moments of comfort, but where he stands at times of challenge and controversy."**

King, Martin Luther Jr. – a minister and civil rights leader who was best known for his nonviolent civil disobedience to combat racial inequality. His 1963 *I Have a Dream* speech during the March on Washington is considered one of the most significant in United States history. He was awarded the Nobel Peace Prize in 1964. (1929-1968)

744. **"To be kind is to respond with sensitivity and human warmth to the hopes and needs of others. Even the briefest touch of kindness can lighten a heavy heart. Kindness can change the lives of people."**

Kyi, Aung San Suu – a Burmese politician who was placed under house arrest for nearly 15 years between 1989-2010. During that time, she became one of the world's most prominent political prisoners. She now heads her country as First State Counsellor. (1945-)

745. **"Ask yourself: Have you been kind today? Make kindness your daily modus operandi and change your world."**

Lennox, Annie – a Scottish singer-songwriter who experienced initial success in the 1980s with the Eurhythmics. In the 1990s, she launched her solo career. VH1 named her "The Greatest White Soul Singer Alive," and *Rolling Stone Magazine* included her in "The 100 Greatest Singers of All Time." (1954-)

746. **"The measure of who we are is what we do with what we have."**

Lombardi, Vince – a football coach who is considered one of the best and most successful coaches in history. He led the Green Bay Packers to five NFL Championships in seven years in the 1960s, including winning the first two Super Bowls in 1966 and 1967. The Super Bowl trophy is named in his honor. (1913-1970)

747. ☺ "I have noticed that the people who are late are often so much jollier than the people who have to wait for them."

Lucas, Edward – a prolific English writer who spent his entire career writing for the humorous magazine *Punch*. He was best known for his short essays, but he also wrote biographies, poems, novels, and plays. (1868-1938)

748. "Many years ago, Rudyard Kipling gave an address at McGill University in Montreal. He said one striking thing which deserves to be remembered. Warning the students against an over-concern for money, or position, or glory, he said: "Someday you will meet a man who cares for none of these things. Then you will know how poor you are."

Luccock, Halford – a prominent Methodist minister and professor of Homiletics at Yale's Divinity School. (1885-1961)

749. ☺ "Those are my principles, and if you don't like them... well, I have others."

Marx, Groucho – a comedian and a film and television star. He was a master of quick wit and considered to be one of the best comedians of the modern era. (1890-1977)

750. "People never care how much you know until they know how much you care."

Maxwell, John – an Australian-born Christian author, speaker, leadership expert, and pastor. He has written many books on leadership, including the bestselling books *The 21 Irrefutable Laws of Leadership* and *The 21 Indispensable Qualities of a Leader*. (1947-)

751. "One of the most sincere forms of respect is actually listening to what another has to say."

McGill, Bryant – a thinker, author, and social media influencer who focuses on human potential. He is one of the most virally read online authors with over 12 million subscribers across diferent platforms.

752. ☺ "Character is what emerges from all the little things you were too busy to do yesterday but did anyway."

McLaughlin, Mignon – a journalist and author who began publishing aphorisms in the 1950s. He collected them into three books: *The Neurotic's Notebook*, *The Second Neurotic's Notebook*, and *The Complete Neurotic's Notebook*. (1913-1983)

753. ☺ "What people say, what people do, and what they say they do are entirely different things."

Mead, Margaret – a popular cultural anthropologist, author, and speaker who was active during the 1960s and 1970s. Her insights helped popularize anthropology in the West. (1901-1978)

754. "Integrity means that you are the same in public as you are in private."

Meyer, Joyce – a Christian author, speaker, and televangelist from Missouri. (1943-)

755. ☺ "Civility costs nothing and buys everything."

Montagu, Mary Wortley – an English aristocrat and writer whose writings challenged contemporary social attitudes towards women. (1689-1762)

756. "Character fashions fate."

Nepos – an ancient Roman biographer. (110-25 BC)

757. "I expect to pass through this world but once. Any good, therefore, that I can do or any kindness I can show to any fellow creature, let me do it now. Let me not defer or neglect it for I shall not pass this way again."

Penn, William – an English Quaker, entrepreneur, philosopher, and founder of the Province of Pennsylvania. (1644-1718)

758. ☺ "We judge others by their behavior. We judge ourselves by our intentions."

Percy, Ian – an organizational psychologist who helps companies transform themselves by reaching for their highest potential. He has authored seven books including *Going Deep*, *The Profitable Power of Purpose* and *Make Your Life a Masterpiece*.

759. "What we achieve inwardly will change outer reality."

Plutarch – a Greek biographer and essayist. (45 -120 AD)

760. ☺ "Men are like wine – some turn to vinegar, but the best improve with age."

Pope John XXIII – Angelo Giuseppe Roncalli was one of fourteen children born to a sharecropper family in a village in Lombardy, Italy. He was elected pope at age 76 and served 4 1/2 years before he died of stomach cancer in 1963. He was canonized a saint in the Roman Catholic Church in 2014. (1881-1963)

761.   ☺ "Character is made by what you stand for; reputation by what you fall for."

Quillen, Robert – a journalist and humorist who wrote about his everyday experiences from his home in Fountain Inn, South Carolina. By 1932, his work had appeared in 400 newspapers around the world. (1887-1948)

762.   "I must learn to love the fool in me the one who feels too much, talks too much, takes too many chances, wins sometimes and loses often, lacks self-control, loves and hates, hurts and gets hurt, promises and breaks promises, laughs and cries."

Rubin, Theodore – a psychiatrist, columnist, and author of more than 25 books of fiction and nonfiction. (1923-)

763.   "We have to dare to be ourselves, however frightening or strange that self may prove to be."

Sarton, May – a Belgian-American poet and author whose many works focused on love, loneliness, aging, nature, and self-doubt. (1912-1995)

764.   ☺ "Politeness is to human nature what warmth is to wax."

Schopenhauer, Arthur – a German philosopher whose writings on morality and psychology were very influential in the 19th and 20th centuries. He was one of the first Western philosophers to give recognition to Eastern philosophy. (1788-1860)

765. "Politeness is a way of showing externally the internal regard we have for others. Good manners are the shadows cast by virtues."

Sheen, Fulton – Catholic bishop famous for his preaching and hosting of radio and television shows from 1930-1968. He is recognized as one of the first televangelists. Efforts are underway to have him recognized as a saint by the Catholic Church. (1895-1979)

766. "Kindness is more than deeds. It is an attitude, an expression, a look, a touch. It is anything that lifts another person."

Strait, C. Neil – a religious leader and writer. (1934-2003)

767. "In life you can never be too kind or too fair; everyone you meet is carrying a heavy load. When you go through your day expressing kindness and courtesy to all you meet, you leave behind a feeling of warmth and good cheer, and you help alleviate the burdens everyone is struggling with."

Tracy, Brian – a Canadian-born American motivational speaker and bestselling self-improvement author. He has written more than 70 books. (1944-)

768. "To remain neutral in situations of injustice is to be complicit in that injustice."

Tutu, Desmond – a South African social rights activist and retired Anglican bishop who became famous during the 1980s as an opponent of apartheid and the first black

Archbishop of Cape Town. He was awarded the Nobel Peace Prize in 1984 and the Presidential Medal of Freedom in 2009. (1931-)

769. **"You can have no dominion greater or less than that over yourself."**

Vinci, Leonardo da – known as the "Renaissance Man," his interests included: invention, painting, sculpting, architecture, science, music, mathematics, engineering, literature, anatomy, geology, astronomy, botany, writing, history, and cartography. The *Mona Lisa* and *The Last Supper* are among his most famous works of art. (1452-1519)

770. **"It's important that people know what you stand for. It's equally important that they know what you won't stand for."**

Waldrip, Mary – an author and editor who is best known for her quotes published in the Reader's Digest and The Atlanta Journal-Constitution. She was the author of *Kate's Korner* column in *The Dawson County Advertiser/News*, in Dawsonville, GA for over 30 years. (1914-1988)

771. ☺ **"Unkind people need your kindness the most. They advertise their pain."**

Warren, Rick – an evangelical Christian pastor and author who is the founder and senior pastor of Saddleback Church in Lake Forest, CA, the 8th largest church in the United States. He is a bestselling author of many Christian books and is best known for *The Purpose Driven Life* (2002). (1954-)

772. "Do all the good you can, by all the means you can, in all the ways you can, in all the places you can, at all the times you can, to all the people you can, as long as you ever can."

Wesley, John – an English theologian and a founder of the Methodist movement. (1703-1791)

773. "There may be times when we are powerless to prevent injustice, but there must never be a time when we fail to protest."

Wiesel, Elie – a Romanian-born, Jewish-American professor and political activist who was a Holocaust survivor and the author of 57 books. He was awarded the Nobel Peace Prize in 1986. (1928-2016)

774. "Be more concerned with your character than with your reputation. Your character is what you really are while your reputation is merely what others think you are."

Wooden, John – called the "Wizard of Westwood," he was a legendary basketball coach at UCLA, where they won 10 NCAA national championships in a 12-year period, including a record seven in a row. (1910-2010)

Charity & Kindness

775. "Be of service. Whether you make yourself available to a friend or co-worker, or you make time every month to do volunteer work, there is nothing that harvests more of a feeling of empowerment than being of service to someone in need."

Anderson, Gillian – an American-British film, television and theatre actress, activist, and writer. (1968-)

776. ☺ "Volunteers are not paid — not because they are worthless, but because they are priceless."

Author Unknown

777. "Volunteers are the only human beings on the face of the earth who reflect this nation's compassion, unselfish caring, patience, and just plain loving one another."

Bombeck, Erma – a popular humorist and bestselling author who was known for her newspaper column that described suburban home life. It ran from the mid-1960s until the late 1990s. (1927-1996)

778. "Nobody made a greater mistake than he who did nothing because he could do only a little."

Burke, Edmund – an Irish-British author and political figure. (1729-1797)

779. "Service to a just cause rewards the worker with more real happiness and satisfaction than any other venture of life."

Catt, Carrie Chapman – a women's rights activist who campaigned for the 19th Amendment to the United States Constitution, which gave women the right to vote in 1920. (1859-1947)

780. "To the wrongs that need resistance, To the right that needs assistance, To the future in the distance, Give yourselves."

Catt, Carrie Chapman – a women's rights activist who campaigned for the 19th Amendment to the United States Constitution, which gave women the right to vote in 1920. (1859-1947)

781. "We make a living by what we do, but we make a life by what we give."

Churchill, Winston – a British army officer, politician, and author. He was the Prime Minister of the United Kingdom from 1940-1945 and again from 1951-1955. His strong leadership during WW II, opposing Nazi fascism and air strikes, earned him recognition as one of Great Britain's most admired and influential historical figures. (1874-1965)

782. "You cannot hope to build a better world without improving the individuals. To that end, each of us must work for our own improvement and, at the same time, share a general responsibility for all humanity, our particular duty being to aid those to whom we think we can be most useful."

Curie, Marie – a Polish and naturalized-French physicist and chemist who conducted pioneering research on radioactivity. She was the first woman to receive a Nobel Prize and the first person to receive two. She was also the first woman to become a professor at the University of Paris. (1867-1934)

783. **"You will learn more about the people you work with in three minutes by asking them what they do for nothing, than by working with them for three years in the same team."**

Dixon, Patrick – a British physician, author, and popular futurist. He is Chairman of Global Change, a growth strategy and forecasting company. (1957-)

784. **"Service is the rent we pay for being. It is the very purpose of life and not something you do in your spare time."**

Edelman, Marian Wright – a children's rights activist. (1939-)

785. **"Paul Revere earned his living as a silversmith. But what do we remember him for? His volunteer work. All activism is volunteering in that it's done above and beyond earning a living and deals with what people really care passionately about. Remember, no one gets paid to rebel. All revolutions start with volunteers."**

Ellis, Susan – the President of Energize, Inc., a training, consulting, and publishing firm that specializes in volunteerism. It was founded in Philadelphia in 1977.

786. "Volunteering is so pervasive it's invisible. We take for granted all the things that have been pioneered by concerned, active volunteers."

Ellis, Susan – the President of Energize, Inc., a training, consulting, and publishing firm that specializes in volunteerism. It was founded in Philadelphia in 1977.

787. "Not he who has much is rich, but he who gives much."

Fromm, Erich – a German social psychologist, psychoanalyst, sociologist, philosopher, and author. His book *The Art of Loving* (1956) was an international bestseller. (1900-1980)

788. "True compassion means not only feeling another's pain but also being moved to help relieve it."

Goleman, Daniel – the bestselling author of *Emotional Intelligence* (1995), he is a psychologist, science journalist, former *New York Times* writer and internationally known thought leader.

789. "It's impossible to be involved in all situations, but there's no excuse not to be involved in something, somewhere, somehow, with someone. Make an ounce of difference."

Goodrich, Richelle – an author, novelist, and poet who writes for young adults. Her writing includes "fantasies, adventures, and some realities, always with a touch of romance." (1968-)

790. "Without community service, we would not have a strong quality of life. It's important to the person

who serves as well as the recipient. It's the way in which we ourselves grow and develop..."

Height, Dorothy – an African-American civil rights and women's rights activist. She served as president of the National Council of Negro Women for forty years and received both the Presidential Medal of Freedom (1994) and the Congressional Gold Medal (2004). (1912-2010)

791. "The best antidote I know for worry is work. The best cure for weariness is the challenge of helping someone who is even more tired. One of the great ironies of life is this: He or she who serves almost always benefits more than he or she who is served."

Hinckley, Gordon – a religious leader and author who was the 15th President of The Church of Jesus Christ of Latter-day Saints, from 1995 until his death. He received the Presidential Medal of Freedom in 2004 for a lifetime of humanitarian service. (1910-2008)

792. "The heart of a volunteer is not measured in size, but by the depth of the commitment to make a difference in the lives of others."

Hollis, DeAnn – attributed to DeAnn Hollis.

793. ☺ "There is no exercise better for the heart than reaching down and lifting people up."

Holmes Jr., John – a poet and professor of Literature and Modern Poetry at Tufts University for 28 years. (1904-1962)

794. ☺ "If you haven't any charity in your heart, you have the worst kind of heart trouble."

Hope, Bob – a comedian, actor, and author whose career spanned nearly 80 years. He appeared in over 70 films, hosted the Academy Awards 19 times (more than any other host), and was the author of 14 books. The song "Thanks for the Memories" is considered his signature song. (1903-2003)

795. **"If you are feeling helpless, help someone."**

Kyi, Aung San Suu – a Burmese politician who was placed under house arrest for nearly 15 years between 1989-2010. During that time, she became one of the world's most prominent political prisoners. She now heads her country as First State Counsellor. (1945-)

796. **"Holding on to anger, resentment and hurt only gives you tense muscles, a headache and a sore jaw from clenching your teeth. Forgiveness gives you back the laughter and the lightness in your life."**

Lunden, Joan – a journalist, author, and television host. She was co-host of ABC's *Good Morning America* from 1980-1997. (1950-)

797. **"Allow the way to your great work to be guided by your service to others."**

Marti, Mollie – a resilience researcher and expert in community crisis recovery and resilience building. Her THRIVE Model of Community Resilience™ assists community-based crisis response, intervention, and positive human development.

798. **"Give out what you most want to come back."**

Sharma, Robin – Canadian self-help writer and leadership speaker. He is best known for *The Monk Who Sold His Ferrari* series. (1965-)

799. "You have not lived a perfect day, even though you have earned your money, unless you have done something for someone, who will never be able to repay you."

Smeltzer, Ruth – a health care provider. (1961-)

800. "I slept and dreamt that life was joy. I awoke and saw that life was service. I acted and behold, service was joy."

Tagore, Rabindranath – an Indian intellectual who strongly influenced Bengali art, literature, and music in the late 19th and early 20th centuries. In 1913, he became the first non-European to win the Nobel Prize in Literature. (1861-1941)

801. "There are two ways of exerting one's strength: one is pushing down, the other is pulling up."

Washington, Booker T. – an African-American leader, educator, and author who came from the last generation of black leaders born into slavery. From 1890-1915, he was a prominent leader in the African-American community. His autobiography *Up From Slavery* (1901) became a bestseller. (1856-1915)

Contentment, Patience & Peace

802. ☺ "The world always looks brighter from behind a smile."

Author Unknown

803. **"Peace comes from within. Do not seek it without."**

Buddha – the "enlightened one" from northeastern India. He was a spiritual teacher and the founder of Buddhism. (563-483 BC)

804. **"The quest for peace begins in the home, in the school and in the workplace."**

Cartwright, Silvia – she became the first female Chief District Court Judge in New Zealand in 1989 and was appointed Governor-General of New Zealand from 2001-2006. (1943-)

805. **"What are you accepting that would not be a part of your ideal day?"**

Cohen, Alan – a popular inspirational author, columnist, and radio show host. (1954-)

806. **"Both what you run from and what you yearn for are within you."**

de Mello, Anthony – a Catholic priest from India who also was a psychotherapist, spiritual teacher, and author. He is well known for his storytelling, which incorporated mystical traditions from the East and the West. (1931-1987)

807. ☺ **"A smile is a curve that sets everything straight."**

Diller, Phyllis – a stand-up comedian and television personality. (1917-2012)

808. **"Learn to be alone and to like it. There is nothing more freeing and empowering than learning to like your own company."**

Hale, Mandy – *New York Times* bestselling author and speaker who is known around the world as "The Single Woman." She seeks to inspire single women to live their best lives and to never settle for less.

809. ☺ **"If someone is too tired to give you a smile, leave one of your own, because no one needs a smile as much as those who have none to give."**

Hirsch, Samson – a German rabbi whose philosophy had a significant influence on the development of Orthodox Judaism. (1808-1888)

810. ☺ **"Smile, it's free therapy."**

Horton, Douglas – a Protestant clergyman and academic leader who was respected for promoting ecumenical relations among major Protestant denominations. (1891-1968)

811. **"Our freedom can be measured by the number of things we can walk away from."**

Howard, Vernon – a spiritual teacher, author, and philosopher. He began his writing career in the 1940s as an author of humor and children's books. In the 1950s, his focus was on the principles of personal development. In the 1960s, his writing concerned spiritual and psychological growth. (1918-1992)

812. ☺ **"Patience is the ability to idle your motor when you feel like stripping your gears."**

Johnson, Barbara – an author dedicated to helping women in despair with her humor and faith. Her bestselling books including *Plant a Geranium in Your Cranium*, *Living Somewhere Between Estrogen and Death*, and *Stick a Geranium in Your Hat and Be Happy*. (1927-2007)

813. **"First keep the peace within yourself, then you can also bring peace to others."**

Kempis, Thomas a – the Dutch author of *The Imitation of Christ*, which is one of the most well-known Christian devotional books. (1380-1471)

814. **"Mankind must put an end to war before war puts an end to mankind."**

Kennedy, John F. – "JFK" was a politician from Massachusetts who became the 35th President of the United States, from January 1961 until his assassination in November 1963. Prior to becoming President, he served as a Democratic congressman and senator. (1917-1963)

815. **"There is no passion to be found playing small – in settling for a life that is less than the one you are capable of living."**

Mandela, Nelson – a South African anti-apartheid leader who became the country's first black President from 1994-1999. He was sentenced to life in prison in 1962 for attempting to overthrow the apartheid government and served 27 years. During that time, he became a symbol for democracy and social justice throughout the world. (1918-2013)

816. **"Enjoy doing nothing, and you can enjoy doing anything. Enjoy having nothing, and you can enjoy whatever you have."**

Marston, Ralph – an author and publisher of *The Daily Motivator*. His website has provided a new motivational message every Monday through Saturday since 1996.

817. "Thoughts will lead you in circles. Silence will bring you back to your center."

Ogunlaru, Rasheed – a life coach, speaker, and author of *Soul Trader - Putting the Heart Back into Your Business*, *The Gift of Inner Success* and *A Zest for Business*. (1970-)

818. "All man's miseries derive from not being able to sit quietly in a room alone."

Pascal, Blaise – a French inventor, writer, and Christian philosopher. (1623-1662)

819. "There is a criterion by which you can judge whether the thoughts you are thinking and the things you are doing are right for you. The criterion is: Have they brought you inner peace?"

Peace Pilgrim – born Mildred Lisette Norman, she was a spiritual teacher, pacifist, vegetarian activist, and peace activist who became known as the "Peace Pilgrim." From 1953-1981 she walked more than 25,000 miles on a personal pilgrimage for peace. (1908-1981)

820. "True silence is the rest of the mind; it is to the spirit what sleep is to the body, nourishment and refreshment."

Penn, William – an English Quaker, entrepreneur, philosopher, and founder of the Province of Pennsylvania. (1644-1718)

821. "Learn to be silent. Let your quiet mind listen and absorb."

Pythagoras – an ancient Greek philosopher who made significant contributions to mathematics and philosophy. He is best known for the Pythagorean theorem that is named in his honor. (570-495 BC)

822. ☺ "Patience is bitter, but its fruit is sweet."

Rousseau, Jean-Jacques – a Swiss philosopher and developer of modern political and educational thought. (1712-1778)

823. "To experience peace does not mean that your life is always blissful. It means that you are capable of tapping into a blissful state of mind amidst the normal chaos of a hectic life."

Taylor, Jill Bolte – a brain scientist, author, and inspirational speaker. In 1996, at the age of 37, she suffered a massive stroke that led to an 8-year recovery that led to her bestselling book *My Stroke of Insight, A Brain Scientist's Personal Journey* (2006). Her 2008 TED talk was the first to go viral on the Internet. (1959-)

824. "We need quiet time to examine our lives openly and honestly - spending quiet time alone gives your mind an opportunity to renew itself and create order."

Taylor, Susan – an influential African-American writer and journalist. From 1981-2000, she served as editor-in-chief of *Essence*, a magazine for African-American women. (1946-)

825. "Loneliness expresses the pain of being alone and solitude expresses the glory of being alone."

Tillich, Paul – a German-American Christian philosopher

and theologian who is considered to be one of the most influential theologians of the 20th Century. (1886-1965)

826. **"Everything we do is infused with the energy with which we do it. If we're frantic, life will be frantic. If we're peaceful, life will be peaceful. And so, our goal in any situation becomes inner peace."**

Williamson, Marianne – a bestselling author, spiritual teacher, and speaker. She has founded and been involved in a number of humanitarian efforts including Project Angel Food - a meals-on-wheels program that serves homebound people with AIDS in the Los Angeles area. (1952-)

Emotions, Energy & Vitality

827. ☺ **"Blessed are the flexible, for they shall not be bent out of shape."**

Author Unknown

828. ☺ **"Crying relieves pressure on the soul."**

Beta, Toba – a writer and economist who was called "Mister Bond" by *Investor Magazine*. He was the author of *Master of Stupidity*.

829. **"Youthfulness is a measure of the dynamism with which we live, not a measure of our age."**

Deonaraine, Ramesh – an economist, management consultant, and author. He was a recipient of the Emily

Gregory Award for Excellence in Teaching at Barnard College, Columbia University – the only Economics Professor to receive the award in 27 years.

830. ☺ **"Your intellect may be confused, but your emotions will never lie to you."**

Ebert, Roger – an author and film critic who worked for the *Chicago Sun-Times* from 1967 until his death in 2013. In 1975, he became the first film critic to win the Pulitzer Prize for Criticism. Ebert and Gene Siskel co-hosted popular television film review shows where they made the phrase "Two Thumbs Up" commonplace – given when both agreed on a positive review. (1967-2013)

831. ☺ **"The idea is to die young as late as possible."**

Montagu, Ashley – formerly known as Israel Ehrenberg, he was a British-American anthropologist who is credited with popularizing the study of race and gender and their relation to politics. (1905-1999)

832. **"What drains your spirit drains your body. What fuels your spirit fuels your body."**

Myss, Carolyn – (pronounced "mace") an author of five *New York Times* bestsellers who describes herself as a mystic – someone who perceives life through the eyes of the soul. (1952-)

833. ☺ **"The heart does not learn things as quickly as the mind."**

Norris, Kathleen Thompson – a popular novelist and newspaper columnist who was one of the most widely read and highest paid female writers in the United States from 1911-1959. She used fiction to encourage values that promoted marriage, motherhood, and service to others. (1880-1966)

834. ☺ **"Youth has no age."**

Picasso, Pablo – a Spanish artist who spent most of his life in France. He is regarded as one of the greatest and most influential artists of all time. It is estimated that he created more than 50,000 works of art, including: paintings, sculptures, ceramics, drawings, prints, tapestries, and rugs. (1881-1973)

835. **"In anger we should refrain both from speech and action."**

Pythagoras – an ancient Greek philosopher who made significant contributions to mathematics and philosophy. He is best known for the Pythagorean theorem that is named in his honor. (570-495 BC)

836. ☺ **"Each of us makes his own weather, determines the color of the skies in the emotional universe which he inhabits."**

Sheen, Fulton – a Catholic bishop famous for his preaching and hosting of radio and television shows from 1930-1968. He is recognized as one of the first televangelists. Efforts are underway to have him recognized as a saint by the Catholic Church. (1895-1979)

837. ☺ **"It is not the years in your life but the life in your years that counts."**

Stevenson II, Adlai E. – a lawyer, diplomat, and Democratic politician from Illinois. He was admired for his intellect, speaking ability, and leadership. (1900-1965)

838. ☺ "Invite your melancholy outside for a walk. Or read it a poem. Or bake it chocolate chip cookies."

> SunWolf, Dr. – a trial attorney, communications and law professor at Santa Clara University, author, and professional storyteller.

Encouragement & Support

839. ☺ "Sandwich every bit of criticism between two layers of praise."

> Ash, Mary Kay – considered to be one of the most successful female entrepreneurs in American history, she founded Mary Kay Cosmetics in a Dallas, Texas storefront in 1963. By the time of her death, her company had 800,000 representatives in 37 countries and annual sales over $200 million. (1918-2001)

840. "I praise loudly. I blame softly."

> Catherine the Great – the most renowned and longest-ruling female leader of Russia. She was Empress of Russia from 1762-1796. Under her leadership, Russia grew significantly and became recognized as one of Europe's great powers. (1729-1796)

841. "Imitation is the sincerest of flattery."

> Colton, Charles – an English cleric, writer, and collector who was well known for his eccentricities. (1780-1832)

842. ☺ "Praise does wonders for our sense of hearing."

Glasow, Arnold – a humor magazine publisher who authored his first book *Glasow's Gloombusters* at age 92. (1905-1998)

843.   ☺ "Think of everybody you talk to as having a flashing sign on their chest saying: Make me feel special!"

Williams, Art – the founder of A.L. Williams & Associates in 1977, which became Primerica Financial Services in 1991. He built a life insurance empire with a simple philosophy: "Buy Term and Invest the Difference" – getting people to switch from conventional whole-life insurance to term policies. (1942-)

Environment & Nature

844.   "I go to nature to be soothed and healed, and to have my senses put in tune once more."

Burroughs, John – an essayist and naturalist. (1837-1921)

845.   "Those who contemplate the beauty of the Earth find reserves of strength that will endure as long as life lasts."

Carson, Rachel – a marine biologist and conservationist who was instrumental in advancing the global environmental movement. (1907-1964)

846.   ☺ "I love to think of nature as an unlimited broadcasting station, through which God speaks to us every hour, if we will only tune in."

Carver, George Washington – an African-American inventor and botanist who was born into slavery in Missouri. His research focused on alternative crops to cotton, like peanuts and sweet potatoes, to provide better nutrition for farm families and improve their quality of life. (1860s-1943)

847. **"The proper use of science is not to conquer nature but to live in it."**

Commoner, Barry – a biologist, college professor, and politician. He was a leading ecologist and one of the founders of the modern environmental movement. (1917-2012)

848. **"People protect what they love."**

Cousteau, Jacques – a French sea explorer, scientist, conservationist, author, and filmmaker who studied sea life and shared his discoveries with the world. (1910-1997)

849. **"Only when the last tree has been cut down, Only when the last river has been poisoned, Only when the last fish has been caught, Only then will you find that money cannot be eaten."**

Cree Indian Prophecy

850. ☺ **"Modern technology owes ecology an apology."**

Eddison, Alan – Director of Green Earth Affairs headquarters in the Republic of Zimbabwe in southern Africa.

851. **"Conservation is a state of harmony between men and land."**

Leopold, Aldo – an author, scientist, and environmentalist who wrote *A Sand County Almanac*. (1887-1948)

852. "We abuse land because we regard it as a commodity belonging to us. When we see land as a community to which we belong, we may begin to use it with love and respect."

Leopold, Aldo – an author, scientist, and environmentalist who wrote *A Sand County Almanac*. (1887-1948)

853. "Nature nourishes the soul. Our homes will either separate us from nature or connect us to it."

Linn, Denise – a Feng Shui expert and author of 17 books including: *Sacred Space, Soul Coaching*, and her personal memoir *If I Can Forgive, So Can You!* She has been a guest on Oprah, Lifetime, Discovery Channel, BBC TV, NBC, and CBS. (1950-)

854. ☺ "There are no passengers on Spaceship Earth. We are all crew."

McLuhan, Marshall – a Canadian professor, philosopher, and intellectual. His work has influenced the advertising and television industries, and he predicted the World Wide Web 30 years before it was developed. (1911-1980)

855. "In every walk with nature one receives far more than he seeks."

Muir, John – a Scottish-American naturalist, author, environmental philosopher, and early advocate for protecting wilderness areas in the United States. (1838-1914)

856. ☺ **"When one tugs at a single thing in nature, he finds it attached to the rest of the world."**

Muir, John – Scottish-American naturalist, author, environmental philosopher, and early advocate for protecting wilderness areas in the United States. (1838-1914)

857. ☺ **"We do not inherit the earth from our ancestors, we borrow it from our children."**

Native American Proverb

858. **"If we continue to address the issue of the environment where we live as though we're the only species that lives here, we'll create a disaster for ourselves."**

Nelson, Gaylord – a former United States Senator and Governor of Wisconsin who was the founder of Earth Day. (1916-2005)

859. **"The fate of the living planet is the most important issue facing mankind."**

Nelson, Gaylord – a former United States Senator and Governor of Wisconsin who was the founder of Earth Day. (1916-2005)

860. **"The wilderness holds answers to questions man has not yet learned to ask."**

Newhall, Nancy – a photography critic who is best known for writing the text for photographs by Ansel Adams and Edward Weston. She was also an accomplished writer on photography, conservation, and culture. (1908-1974)

861.   ☺ "May your search through nature lead you to yourself."

Park Sign

862.   "Wilderness is not a luxury, but a necessity of the human spirit."

Peaks Foundation

863.   "The activist is not the man who says the river is dirty. The activist is the man who cleans up the river."

Perot, Ross – a businessman and Presidential candidate in 1992 and 1996. He left a position with IBM in 1962 and founded Electronic Data Systems (EDS) in Dallas, TX. In 1984, General Motors bought control of EDS for $2.4 billion. (1930-)

864.   "I think the environment should be put in the category of our national security. Defense of our resources is just as important as defense abroad. Otherwise what is there to defend?"

Redford, Robert – a leading actor, film director, environmentalist, and founder of the Sundance Film Festival. In 2014, *Time Magazine* listed him on their annual Time 100 as one of the Most Influential People in the World. They described him as the "Godfather of Indie Film." (1936-)

865.   "Anything else you're interested in is not going to happen if you can't breathe the air and drink the water. Don't sit this one out. Do something."

Sagan, Carl – a popular astronomer, scientist, and author. (1934-1996)

866. ☺ **"The universe is not required to be in perfect harmony with human ambition."**

Sagan, Carl – a popular astronomer, scientist, and author. (1934-1996)

867. ☺ **"Man is a complex being: he makes deserts bloom – and lakes die."**

Stern, Gil – attributed to Gil Stern.

868. ☺ **"We're in a giant car heading towards a brick wall and everyone's arguing over where they're going to sit."**

Suzuki, David – a Canadian environmental activist and professor from 1963-2001. He is best known for his television and radio programs, documentaries, books about nature and the environment, and for criticizing governments for their lack of environmental protection efforts. (1936-)

869. ☺ **"We are living on this planet as if we had another one to go to."**

Sweringen, Terri – an Ohio nurse who organized protests against Waste Technologies Industries' toxic waste incinerator in East Liverpool, OH. Her actions led to stricter limits for heavy metals and dioxin emissions from waste incinerators and resulted in her receiving the Goldman Environmental Prize in 1997.

870. ☺ "Because we don't think about future generations, they will never forget us."

Tikkanen, Henrik – a Finnish author. (1924-1984)

871. ☺ "Don't blow it – good planets are hard to find."

Time Magazine quote.

872. "Plans to protect air and water, wilderness and wildlife are in fact plans to protect man."

Udall, Stewart – a former Arizona congressman and Secretary of the Interior. (1920-2010)

873. ☺ "Suburbia is where the developer bulldozes out the trees, then names the streets after them."

Vaughan, Bill – a *Kansas City Star* columnist and author. (1915-1977)

874. "I would feel more optimistic about a bright future for man if he spent less time proving that he can outwit Nature and more time tasting her sweetness and respecting her seniority."

White, E. B. – an author of books for children including: *Stuart Little* (1945), *Charlotte's Web* (1952), and *The Trumpet of the Swan* (1970). He also co-authored the classic English language style guide *The Elements of Style*. (1899-1985)

875. ☺ "One planet, one experiment."

Wilson, Edward – a biologist, researcher, naturalist, and author. He is considered the world's leading authority on ants. (1929-)

876. ☺ "If you want to see an endangered species, get up and look in the mirror."

> Young, John – a former astronaut who is the only person to have piloted and commanded four different classes of spacecraft. He made six space flights over 42 years at NASA - the longest career of any astronaut in history. In 1972 he became the ninth person to walk on the Moon. (1930-)

Gratitude

877. "Let gratitude be the pillow upon which you kneel to say your nightly prayer. And let faith be the bridge you build to overcome evil and welcome good."

> Angelou, Maya – an African-American poet, author, and civil rights activist. (1928-2014)

878. "Gratitude makes sense of our past, brings peace for today, and creates a vision for tomorrow."

> Beattie, Melody – an author of self-help books on co-dependent relationships. (1948-)

879. "Gratitude unlocks the fullness of life. It turns what we have into enough, and more. It turns denial into acceptance, chaos to order, confusion to clarity. It can turn a meal into a feast, a house into a home, a stranger into a friend."

> Beattie, Melody – an author of self-help books on co-dependent relationships. (1948-)

880. "Someone's sitting in the shade today because someone planted a tree a long time ago."

Buffett, Warren – a businessman and investor who is one of the wealthiest and most influential people in the world. He is CEO of Berkshire Hathaway and known throughout the world for his philanthropic efforts. (1930-)

881. "Gratitude helps you to grow and expand; gratitude brings joy and laughter into your life and into the lives of all those around you."

Caddy, Eileen – a spiritual teacher and New Age author. (1917-2006)

882. ☺ "When it comes to life the critical thing is whether you take things for granted or take them with gratitude."

Chesterton, G. K. – a prolific English writer who wrote 80 books, hundreds of poems and short stories, 4,000 essays, and several plays. He was also a poet, philosopher, Catholic lay theologian, and biographer. (1874-1936)

883. "Appreciation can change a day, even change a life. Your willingness to put it into words is all that is necessary."

Cousins, Margaret – an Irish-Indian educator who moved to India in 1915 at age 37. She is credited with composing the tune for the Indian National Anthem "Jana Gana Mana" in 1919, and for establishing the All India Women's Conference (AIWC) in 1927. (1878-1954)

884. "If the only prayer you said was thank you, that would be enough."

Eckhart, Meister – a German theologian and mystic who was a member of the Dominicans religious order. (1260-1328)

885. ☺ **"If you were going to die soon and had only one phone call to make, who would you call and what would you say? And why are you waiting?"**

Levine, Stephen – a poet, author, and spiritual teacher who is best known for his work on death and dying. He made the teachings of Theravada Buddhism more popular in the West. His works often referenced a creator, which differentiated his teaching from other contemporary Buddhist writers. (1937-2016)

886. **"If you are really thankful, what do you do? You share."**

Stone, W. Clement – a successful businessman, philanthropist, and self-help book author. He was a high school dropout and a rags-to-riches success story. In 1919, he created the Combined Insurance Company of America, which had more than $1 billion in assets by 1979. (1902-2002)

887. ☺ **"Feeling gratitude and not expressing it is like wrapping a present and not giving it."**

Ward, William – one of America's most quoted writers of inspirational sayings. He is the author of *Fountains of Faith*. (1921-1994)

888. **"Be thankful for what you have; you'll end up having more. If you concentrate on what you don't have, you will never, ever have enough."**

Winfrey, Oprah – one of the richest and most influential women in the world. She is a media mogul, television talk show host, actress, producer, and philanthropist. *The Oprah Winfrey Show* aired from 1986-2011. She was awarded the Presidential Medal of Freedom in 2013. (1954-)

Happiness & Joy

889. ☺ **"Life itself is the proper binge."**

Child, Julia – a popular chef, author, and television personality who introduced French cuisine to the American public with her cookbook *Mastering the Art of French Cooking*. Her television show *The French Chef* debuted in 1963. (1912-2004)

890. **"You will never be happier than you expect. To change your happiness, change your expectation."**

Davis, Bette – an actress of film, television, and theater. She is considered one of the greatest actresses in Hollywood history. (1908-1989)

891. **"Your body cannot heal without play. Your mind cannot heal without laughter. Your soul cannot heal without joy."**

Fenwick, Catherine Rippenger – a Canadian author, educator, therapist, and well-known speaker. She has written for several journals, magazines, and newspapers. Her three published books include: *Love and Laughter: A Healing Journey* (2004), *Telling My Sister's Story* (1996), and *Healing With Humour* (1995).

892. "We have overstretched our personal boundaries and forgotten that true happiness comes from living an authentic life fueled with a sense of purpose and balance."

Hall, Kathleen – an expert on stress, mindful living, and mindfulness who is the founder of the Stress Institute and the Mindful Living Network. She started her career in finance on Wall Street, before deciding to leave corporate stress behind. Martha Stewart named her the "Stress Queen." (1951-)

893. ☺ "Sometimes your joy is the source of your smile, but sometimes your smile can be the source of your joy."

Hanh, Thich Nhat – a Vietnamese Zen Buddhist monk, teacher, author, poet, and peace activist. (1926-)

894. ☺ "We don't laugh because we're happy – we're happy because we laugh."

James, William – a philosopher and psychologist who was one of the leading thinkers of the late 19th century. He is considered to be one of America's most influential philosophers and is often referred to as the "Father of Psychology." (1842-1910)

895. ☺ "You can be right, or you can be happy."

Jampolsky, Gerald – an inspirational speaker and author who is an authority in the fields of psychiatry, health, business, and education. He is the founder of The Center for Attitudinal Healing, which has 130 satellite centers around the world. (1925-)

896. "He who smiles rather than rages is always the stronger."

Japanese Wisdom

897. ☺ "Most folks are about as happy as they make up their minds to be."

Lincoln, Abraham – a politician and lawyer who became the 16th President of the United States, from 1861 until his assassination in 1865. He led the country during the Civil War, preserving the Union, abolishing slavery, and strengthening the federal government. (1809-1865)

898. "The biggest human temptation is to settle for too little."

Merton, Thomas – a Catholic writer, social activist, and Trappist monk at the Abbey of Gethsemane in Kentucky, where he lived for 27 years. He is considered the most influential American Catholic author of the 20th century and was a strong supporter of the nonviolent civil rights and peace movements. In later life, he became very interested in Asian religions. The Dalai Lama said that Merton had a more profound understanding of Buddhism than any other Christian he had known. (1915-1968)

899. "Every time you smile at someone, it is an action of love, a gift to that person, a beautiful thing."

Mother Teresa – a Catholic nun who founded the Missionaries of Charity religious order and devoted her life to caring for the poor in the streets of Kolkata, India and eventually all over the world. She founded the Missionaries of Charity in 1950, which grew to more than 4,500 sisters in 133 countries by 2012. Members of the congregation take vows of chastity, poverty, obedience and a fourth vow: to give "wholehearted free service to the poorest of the poor." She was canonized as a saint of the Catholic Church in 2016. (1910-1997)

900. ☺ **"Happiness doesn't come from doing what we like to do but from liking what we have to do."**

Peterson, Wilferd – an author and advertising executive from Grand Rapids, MI. He has authored nine books and written articles for popular magazines. (1900-1995)

901. **"It is of the small joys and little pleasures that the greatest of our days are built."**

Radmacher, Mary – an author, artist, and professional speaker. She is the author *of Lean Forward into Your Life* (2007) and *Live Boldly.* (2008)

902. ☺ **"Happiness is not a state to arrive at, but a manner of traveling."**

Runbeck, Margaret Lee – an author of 16 books on spiritual and inspirational topics. (1905-1956)

903. ☺ **"Happiness is nothing more than good health and a bad memory."**

Schweitzer, Albert – a theologian, philosopher, physician, and medical missionary in Africa. He earned a Nobel Peace Prize in 1952. (1875-1965)

904. **"Look at everything as though you were seeing it for the first or the last time, then your time on earth will be filled with glory."**

Smith, Betty – born Elisabeth Wehner, she was an author who is best known for her book *A Tree Grows in Brooklyn.* (1896-1972)

905. "It is not how much we have, but how much we enjoy that makes happiness."

Spurgeon, Charles – a British Baptist preacher who was known as the "Prince of Preachers." (1834-1892)

906. ☺ "Nothing you wear is more important than your smile."

Stevens, Connie – an actress and singer. (1938-)

907. ☺ "If only we'd stop trying to be happy we'd have a pretty good time."

Wharton, Edith – a novelist and short story writer who was nominated for the Nobel Prize in Literature in 1927, 1928, and 1930. (1862-1937)

908. ☺ "Some cause happiness wherever they go; others whenever they go."

Wilde, Oscar – Irish playwright, novelist, essayist and poet who became one of London's most popular playwrights in the early 1890s. He is well known for his witty sayings, his *novel The Picture of Dorian Gray*, his plays, and the circumstances surrounding his imprisonment and early death. (1854-1900)

Hope & Optimism

909. ☺ "It is never too late to be what you might have been."

Eliot, George – the penname of British writer Mary Ann Evans who was an English novelist, poet, journalist, and one of the leading writers of the Victorian era. (1819-1880)

910. ☺ **"Today, you have 100% of your life left."**

Hopkins, Tom – a motivational speaker, trainer, and author who has dedicated his professional life to training and inspiring people to achieve their highest potential.

This quote is also attributed to Tom Landry, one of the most successful coaches in National Football League (NFL) history. He was the head coach of the Dallas Cowboys for 29-years. During that time, they enjoyed 20 consecutive winning seasons and won two Super Bowls. His 250 career head coaching wins rank him third in NFL history (only Don Shula's 328 wins and George Halas's 318 wins rank higher). (1924-2000)

911. **"The best way to not feel hopeless is to get up and do something. Don't wait for good things to happen to you. If you go out and make some good things happen, you will fill the world with hope, you will fill yourself with hope."**

Obama, Barack – the 44th President of the United States and the first African-American to be elected President from 2009-2017. He was born in Hawaii, attended Columbia University and Harvard Law School, and worked as a community organizer, civil rights attorney, and law professor before entering politics. From 1997-2004, he served as an Illinois State Senator and then served in United States Senate from 2005-2008. (1961-)

Love

912. ☺ "Pursue what catches your heart, not what catches your eyes."

> Bennett, Roy – a thought leader who shares positive thoughts and creative insight in his writings. He is the author of *The Light in the Heart*."

913. "Judge nothing, you will be happy. Forgive everything, you will be happier. Love everything, you will be happiest."

> Chinmoy, Sri – an Indian spiritual leader who taught meditation in the West after moving to New York City in 1964. He was a prolific author, artist, poet, and musician who held public events focused on inner peace. (1931-2007)

914. "When we feel love and kindness toward others, it not only makes others feel loved and cared for, but it helps us also to develop inner happiness and peace."

> Dalai Lama – the 14th Dalai Lama who functions as the spiritual leader of Tibet. He describes himself as a simple Buddhist monk. Born to a farming family in northeastern Tibet, he was recognized as the reincarnation of the 13th Dalai Lama at the age of two. (1935-)

915. "I grasped the meaning of the greatest secret that human poetry and human thought and belief have to impart: The salvation of man is through love and in love."

> Frankl, Viktor - an Austrian neurologist and psychiatrist who was a Holocaust survivor. His bestselling book,

Man's Search for Meaning, shares his concentration camp experiences, which led him to discover the importance of finding a reason to continue living in even the most brutal conditions. (1905-1997)

916. **"I believe that imagination is stronger than knowledge. That myth is more potent than history. That dreams are more powerful than facts. That hope always triumphs over experience. That laughter is the only cure for grief. And I believe that love is stronger than death."**

Fulghum, Robert – the author of *All I Really Need to Know I Learned in Kindergarten*. (1937-)

917. **"Where we love is home - home that our feet may leave, but not our hearts."**

Holmes Sr., Oliver Wendell – a physician, poet, and author who is considered to be one of the best writers of his time. (1809-1894)

918. **"I have never met a person whose greatest need was anything other than real, unconditional love. You can find it in a simple act of kindness toward someone who needs help. There is no mistaking love...it is the common fiber of life, the flame that heats our soul, energizes our spirit and supplies passion to our lives."**

Kubler-Ross, Elisabeth – a Swiss-American psychiatrist and pioneer in near-death studies who authored *On Death and Dying* in 1997. (1926-2004)

919. "Love doesn't just sit there, like a stone; it has to be made, like bread, remade all the time, made new."

Le Guin, Ursula – an author of fantasy and science fiction novels, children's books, and short stories. (1929-)

920. "Do not waste time bothering whether you "love" your neighbor; act as if you did. As soon as we do this we find one of the great secrets. When you are behaving as if you loved someone you will presently come to love him."

Lewis, C. S. – an Irish-born novelist and lay theologian who is well known for his fictional works like *The Screwtape Letters* and *The Chronicles of Narnia*, and for his non-fiction books including *Mere Christianity* and *Miracles*. (1898-1963)

921. "We may give without loving, but we cannot love without giving."

Meltzer, Bernard – an advice call-in radio show host of *What's Your Problem?* in Philadelphia, from 1967 to the mid-1990s. (1916-1998)

922. "It is not how much you do, but how much love you put in the doing."

Mother Teresa – a Catholic nun who founded the Missionaries of Charity religious order and devoted her life to caring for the poor in the streets of Kolkata, India and eventually all over the world. She founded the Missionaries of Charity in 1950, which grew to more than 4,500 sisters in 133 countries by 2012. Members of the congregation take vows of chastity, poverty, obedience and a fourth vow: to give "wholehearted free service to the poorest of the poor." She was canonized as a saint of the Catholic Church in 2016. (1910-1997)

923. "People who are lonely and depressed are three to 10 times more likely to get sick and die prematurely than those who have a strong sense of love and community. I don't know any other single factor that affects our health - for better and for worse - to such a strong degree."

Ornish, Dean – a physician, researcher, bestselling author, professor, and founder and president of the nonprofit Preventive Medicine Research Institute. He is well known for his promotion of healthy diets and lifestyle changes to control coronary artery disease and other chronic diseases. Learn more at www.ornish.com. (1953-)

924. ☺ "Love is like an hourglass, with the heart filling up as the brain empties."

Renard, Jules – a French author and philosopher. (1864-1910)

925. ☺ "Love is friendship set on fire."

Taylor, Jeremy – a cleric in the Church of England who is considered one of the greatest English prose writers. He is referred to as the "Shakespeare of Divines" for his poetic style of writing. (1613-1667)

926. "The first duty of love is to listen."

Tillich, Paul – a German-American Christian philosopher and theologian who is considered to be one of the most influential theologians of the 20th Century. (1886-1965)

927. "Time is too slow for those who wait, too swift for those who fear, too long for those who grieve, too short for those who rejoice, but for those who love, time is eternity."

Van Dyke Jr., Henry – an author, educator, and clergyman. He was appointed by President Woodrow Wilson to be Minister to the Netherlands and Luxembourg in 1913. He was also a close friend of Helen Keller, who wrote of him, "Dr. Van Dyke is the kind of a friend to have when one is up against a difficult problem. He will take trouble, days and nights of trouble, if it is for somebody else or for some cause he is interested in." (1852-1933)

928. ☺ "Many who have spent a lifetime in it can tell us less of love than the child that lost a dog yesterday."

Wilder, Thornton – a playwright and novelist who won three Pulitzer Prizes for the novel *The Bridge of San Luis Rey* and two plays: *Our Town* and *The Skin of Our Teeth*. (1897-1975)

Meaning & Purpose

929. ☺ "Life is not measured by the number of breaths we take, but by the moments that take our breath away."

Author Unknown

930. ☺ "You may be only one person in this world, but to one person at one time, you are the world."

Author Unknown

931. "Life can be long or short, it all depends on how you choose to live it. It's like forever, always changing. For any of us our forever could end in an hour, or a hundred years from now. You can never know for sure, so you'd better make every second count. What you have to decide is how you want your life to be. If your forever was ending tomorrow, is this how you'd want to have spent it?"

Dessen, Sarah – a bestselling author who often writes about the changes that young people go through when they experience tragedy or loss, as well as the way that personality changes over time. (1970-)

932. ☺ "If we would only give, just once, the same amount of reflection to what we want to get out of life that we give to the question of what to do with a two weeks' vacation, we would be startled at our false standards and the aimless procession of our busy days."

Fisher, Dorothy Canfield – an educational reformer, social activist, and bestselling author. She was a strong supporter of women's rights, racial equality, and lifelong education. (1879-1958)

933. "Those who have a 'why' to live, can bear with almost any 'how'."

Frankl, Viktor – an Austrian neurologist and psychiatrist who was a Holocaust survivor. His bestselling book, *Man's Search for Meaning*, shares his concentration camp experiences that led him to discover the importance of finding a reason to continue living in even the worst of conditions. (1905-1997)

934. ☺ **"Men for the sake of getting a living forget to live."**

Fuller, Margaret – a journalist and women's rights advocate. (1810-1850)

935. **"It is more noble to give yourself completely to one individual than to labor diligently for the salvation of the masses."**

Hammarskjold, Dag – a Swedish diplomat, economist, and author. He was the second secretary-general of the United Nations, from 1953 until his death in a 1961 plane crash. In recognition of his leadership and many accomplishments, President John F. Kennedy called him "the greatest statesman of our century." (1905-1961)

936. **"If a man hasn't discovered something that he will die for, he isn't fit to live."**

King, Martin Luther Jr. – a minister and civil rights leader who was best known for his nonviolent civil disobedience to combat racial inequality. His 1963 *I Have a Dream* speech, during the March on Washington, is considered to be one of the most significant in United States history. He was awarded the Nobel Peace Prize in 1964. (1929-1968)

937. ☺ **"It is good to have an end to journey towards, but it is the journey that matters in the end."**

Le Guin, Ursula – an author of fantasy and science fiction novels, children's books, and short stories. (1929-)

938. ☺ **"Even if I knew that tomorrow the world would go to pieces, I would still plant my apple tree."**

Luther, Martin – a German priest and theologian who led the Protestant Reformation, which rejected many of the teachings and practices of the Roman Catholic Church. (1483-1546)

939. ☺ **"The measure of life (, after all,) is not its duration, but its donation."**

Attributed to both Peter Marshall and Corrie Ten Boom.

Peter Marshall – a Scottish-American preacher who was pastor of the New York Avenue Presbyterian Church in Washington, DC and twice served as Chaplain of the United States Senate. (1902-1949)

Corrie Ten Boom – the first licensed female watchmaker in the Netherlands. She and her Christian family helped many Jews escape the Nazi Holocaust during WW II, which led to her being sent to a concentration camp. Her life story is told in the famous book and movie, *The Hiding Place*. (1892-1983)

940. ☺ **"Love is only a dirty trick played on us to achieve continuation of the species."**

Maugham, William – a British playwright, novelist, and short story writer. He was among the most popular and highest paid writers during the 1930s. (1874-1965)

941. **"We all die. The goal isn't to live forever, the goal is to create something that will."**

Palahniuk, Chuck – a novelist who is well known as the author of *Fight Club*. His writings are often considered dark and disturbing. (1962-)

942. **"Live with intention. Walk to the edge. Listen hard. Practice wellness. Play with abandon. Laugh. Choose**

with no regret. Appreciate your friends. Continue to learn. Do what you love. Live as if this is all there is."

Radmacher, Mary – an author, artist, and professional speaker. She is the author of *Lean Forward into Your Life* (2007) and *Live Boldly*. (2008)

943. "Humankind has not woven the web of life. We are but one thread within it. Whatever we do to the web, we do to ourselves. All things are bound together. All things connect."

Seattle, Chief – a Native American leader who was a chief of the Suquamish Tribe. The city of Seattle is named after him. (1786-1866)

944. ☺ "Life is not a matter of having good cards, but of playing a poor hand well."

Stevenson, Robert Louis – a Scottish novelist who authored *Treasure Island*. (1850-1894)

945. "It is not enough to be busy. So are the ants. The question is: What are we busy about?"

Thoreau, Henry – an essayist, poet, philosopher, abolitionist, naturalist, surveyor, and historian. He is best known for his book *Walden*, which was his reflection on living simply in nature. His writings laid the foundation for modern-day environmentalism. (1817-1862)

946. "The purpose of life is to discover your gift. The work of life is to develop it. The meaning of life is to give your gift away."

Viscott, David – a psychiatrist, author, businessman, and

media personality. He was a professor of psychiatry at UCLA and was one of the first psychiatrists to do a talk radio show, where he offered psychological counseling to on-air patients. (1938-1996)

Meditation, Prayer & Reflection

947. ☺ "Don't ask for a light load, but rather ask for a strong back."

Author Unknown

948. "Inside myself is a place where I live all alone and that's where you renew your springs that never dry up."

Buck, Pearl – a writer who spent the first 42 years of her life in China. She was the first woman to win the Nobel Prize for Literature and became a prominent advocate for the rights of women and minority groups. (1892-1973)

949. ☺ "I prayed for twenty years but received no answer until I prayed with my legs."

Douglass, Frederick – one of the most influential African-Americans of the 19th Century. He was known as a convincing speaker and writer who was devoted to ending slavery and winning equal rights for African-Americans. (1818-1895)

950. "Follow effective action with quiet reflection. From the quiet reflection will come even more effective action."

Drucker, Peter – an Austrian-born American management consultant, educator, and author. He has been called the "Founder of Modern Management." (1909-2005)

951. ☺ **"Pray as if God will take care of all; act as if all is up to you."**

Ignatius of Loyola – a Spanish priest, theologian, and founder of the Society of Jesus religious order, commonly known as the Jesuits. Their ministry is focused on education in schools, colleges, universities, seminaries, and on research-based pursuits. (1491-1556)

952. **"Meditation is not a means to an end. It is both the means and the end."**

Krishnzmurti, Jiddhu – an Indian philosopher, speaker, and writer. His writings focused on bringing about a radical change in society. (1895-1986)

953. **"The soul always knows what to do to heal itself. The challenge is to silence the mind."**

Myss, Carolyn – (pronounced "mace") an author of five *New York Times* bestsellers who describes herself as a mystic – someone who perceives life through the eyes of the soul. (1952-)

954. ☺ **"At the end of the day, I can end up just totally wacky, because I've made mountains out of molehills. With meditation, I can keep them as molehills."**

Starr, Ringo – born Richard Starkey, he is an English drummer, singer, and songwriter who is most famous for being the drummer of the Beatles. He is recognized as one of the greatest drummers of all time and was inducted into the Rock and Roll Hall of Fame as both a Beatle and a solo artist. (1940-)

955. **"Thank you is the best prayer that anyone could say. I say that one a lot. Thank you expresses extreme gratitude, humility, understanding."**

Walker, Alice – a writer, poet, and activist who wrote the Pulitzer Prize winning novel *The Color Purple*. (1944-)

Pets

956. ☺ **"My goal in life is to become as wonderful as my dog thinks I am."**

Buxbaum, Martin – a poet and author whose works include: *Rivers of Thought*, *Whispers in the Wind* and *The Underside of Heaven*. (1912-1991)

957. ☺ **"Dogs have given us their absolute all. We are the center of their universe, we are the focus of their love and faith and trust. They serve us in return for scraps. It is without a doubt the best deal man has ever made."**

Caras, Roger – a wildlife photographer, preservationist, writer, and television personality. (1928-2001)

958. ☺ **"Time spent with cats is never wasted."**

Freud, Sigmund – an Austrian neurologist and the founder of psychoanalysis. (1856-1939)

959. ☺ "No man knows a truer love or loyalty, than a dog he has shared his heart with."

Paige, Colleen – a pet and family lifestyle expert who is the creator of National Dog Day, National Cat Day and other pet celebration days. She is the author of *The Good Behavior Book For Dogs*.

960. ☺ "No man can be condemned for owning a dog. As long as he has a dog, he has a friend."

Rogers, Will – a humorist, actor, and social commentator. (1879-1935)

961. ☺ "There are two means of refuge from the miseries of life: music and cats."

Schweitzer, Albert – a theologian, philosopher, physician, and medical missionary in Africa. He earned a Nobel Peace Prize in 1952. (1875-1965)

962. ☺ "A dog is the only thing on earth that loves you more than you love yourself."

Shaw, Henry – using the penname, "Josh Billings," he was a famous humor writer and lecturer, second only to Mark Twain in the late 1800s. (1818-1885)

963. ☺ "There is no psychiatrist in the world like a puppy licking your face."

Williams, Bernard – an English professor, moral philosopher, and author. He was known for his efforts to realign the study of moral philosophy to psychology, history, and the Greeks. He was a Professor of Philosophy at Cambridge and the University of California, Berkeley, and was knighted in 1999. (1929-2003)

Relationships

964. ☺ "Seeing ourselves as others see us would probably confirm our worst suspicions about them."

Adams, Franklin – a witty newspaper columnist and radio personality. (1881-1960)

965. "A faithful friend is a strong defense; And he that hath found him hath found a treasure."

Alcott, Louisa May – a novelist and poet who is best known as the author of *Little Women*. (1832-1888)

966. ☺ "Friendship isn't a big thing – it's a million little things."

Author Unknown

967. "The bond that links your true family is not one of blood, but of respect and joy in each other's life."

Bach, Richard – an author of popular 1970s bestsellers and numerous works of fiction and non-fiction. (1936-)

968. "A life is measured by the roads we travel and the people we share it with. This is how we grow. This is how we add light to the world."

Basheer, Adele – Adele and Jamie Basheer are a South Australian couple who have a simple vision to make a positive difference in the world by touching people's hearts through their greeting card business.

969. ☺ "Spend some time this weekend on home improvement; improve your attitude toward your family."

Bennett, Bo – a businessman, author, motivational speaker, and amateur comedian. (1972-)

970. "Life appears to me too short to be spent in nursing animosity or registering wrongs."

Bronte, Charlotte – an English novelist and poet whose most famous work was the literary classic *Jane Eyre*. (1816-1855)

971. ☺ "Happiness is having a large, loving, caring, close-knit family – in another city."

Burns, George – a comedian and actor who was one of the few entertainers who experienced success over 75 years - spanning vaudeville, radio, movies, and television. He and wife, Gracie Allen, formed the comedy duo of Burns and Allen. In 1977, at the age of 81, he played the role of God in the hit movie *Oh, God!* (1896-1996)

972. ☺ "You can make more friends in two months by becoming interested in other people than you can in two years by trying to get other people interested in you."

Carnegie, Dale – a writer and lecturer who developed popular courses on self-improvement. His book *How to Win Friends and Influence People* was published in 1936. It has sold over 30 million copies and is still popular today. (1888-1955)

973. ☺ "My love, there is no plan B."

Carstairs, Melody – an Australian life coach, personal trainer, fitness competitor, and judge. She is also a business entrepreneur in the health and fitness industry.

974. ☺ "The most important things in life aren't things."

D'Angelo, Anthony – an educational entrepreneur who founded Collegiate EmPowerment. He has dedicated his life to helping young adults to create a life worth living. (1972-)

975. ☺ "I looked up my family tree and found out I was the sap."

Dangerfield, Rodney – a stand-up comedian, actor, producer, and writer. He was known for the catchphrase "I don't get no respect!" His 1980s film roles include: *Easy Money*, *Caddyshack*, and *Back to School*. (1921-2004)

976. "When you start about family, about lineage and ancestry, you are talking about every person on earth."

Haley, Alex – an author best known for *Roots: The Saga of a Family* and *The Autobiography of Malcolm X*. (1921-1992)

977. ☺ "A friend is one who knows you and loves you just the same."

Hubbard, Elbert – a writer, publisher, artist, and philosopher who was an influential supporter of the Arts and Crafts Movement. He died aboard the British ocean liner, RMS Lusitania, when it was sunk by a German submarine off the coast of Ireland on May 7, 1915. (1856-1915)

978. ☺ "Never cut what you can untie."

Joubert, Joseph – a French moralist and essayist who is best known for his *Pensées* (Collected Thoughts), which were published after his death. (1754-1824)

979. ☺ "Be not angry that you cannot make others as you wish them to be, since you cannot make yourself as you wish to be."

Kempis, Thomas a – the Dutch author of *The Imitation of Christ*, which is one of the most well-known Christian devotional books. (1380-1471)

980. ☺ "To handle yourself, use your head; to handle others, use your heart."

Laird, Donald – author of *Sizing Up People* (1964) and other books on personal and professional development. (1897-1969)

981. "You never really understand a person until you consider things from his point of view."

Lee, Harper – the author of the literary classic *To Kill a Mockingbird* (1960). (1926-2016)

982. "If you want to make peace with your enemy, you have to work with your enemy. Then he becomes your partner."

Mandela, Nelson – a South African anti-apartheid leader who became the country's first black President from 1994-1999. He was sentenced to life in prison in 1962 for attempting to overthrow the apartheid government and served 27 years. During that time, he became a symbol for democracy and social justice throughout the world. (1918-2013)

983. **"When you choose your friends, don't be short-changed by choosing personality over character."**

Maugham, William – a British playwright, novelist, and short story writer. He was among the most popular and highest paid writers during the 1930s. (1874-1965)

984. ☺ **"We teach people how to treat us."**

McGraw, Phil – a psychologist, author, and television host. He is one of the best-known mental health professionals in the world. Known for making complicated information easy to understand, his *Dr. Phil* talk show is one of the top-rated programs on daytime television. (1950-)

985. **"I was born to a woman I never knew and raised by another who took in orphans. I do not know my background, my lineage, my biological or cultural heritage. But when I meet someone new, I treat them with respect... For after all, they could be my people."**

Michener, James – a bestselling author of more than 40 books. His long works of historical fiction cover many generations in specific geographic locations. His bestsellers: *Hawaii*, *Alaska*, *Texas*, and *Poland* are examples of this. (1907-1997)

986. ☺ **"To keep your marriage brimming, With love in the loving cup, Whenever you're wrong, admit it; Whenever you're right, shut up."**

Nash, Ogden – a poet about whom the *New York Times* remarked, his "droll verse with its unconventional rhymes made him the country's best-known producer of humorous poetry." His most notable work was published in 14 volumes between 1931-1972. (1902-1971)

987. **"When we know ourselves to be connected to all others, acting compassionately is simply the natural thing to do."**

Remen, Rachel – a physician and author who has suffered from Crohn's disease for most of her life. She was a pioneer of Holistic and Integrative Medicine. Her curriculum for medical students, called *The Healer's Art*, offers the wisdom of both doctor and patient and is taught in 90 American medical schools. (1938-)

988. **"The quality of your life is the quality of your relationships."**

Robbins, Tony – a popular self-help author and motivational speaker. His bestselling books include: *Unlimited Power* (1986), *Awaken the Giant Within* (1991) and *Money: Master the Game* (2014). (1960-)

989. ☺ **"It takes a great deal of bravery to stand up to our enemies, but just as much to stand up to our friends."**

Rowling, J.K. – a novelist and author of the *Harry Potter* series, one of the most popular book and film series in history. At one point in her life, she was a welfare recipient. Today, she is one of the wealthiest women in the world. (1965-)

990. ☺ **"Before I met my husband, I'd never fallen in love. I'd stepped in it a few times."**

Rudner, Rita – a comedian and actress who began her career as a Broadway dancer. The lack of women stand-up comics led her to change careers in her mid-20s. Her popularity spread with appearances on the *Tonight Show with Johnny Carson* and comedy specials on HBO. (1953-)

991. ☺ **"When I eventually met Mr. Right I had no idea that his first name was Always."**

Rudner, Rita – a comedian and actress who began her career as a Broadway dancer. The lack of women stand-up comics led her to change careers in her mid-20s. Her popularity spread with appearances on the *Tonight Show with Johnny Carson* and comedy specials on HBO. (1953-)

992. **"Silences make the real conversations between friends. Not the saying but the never needing to say is what counts."**

Runbeck, Margaret Lee – an author of 16 books on spiritual and inspirational topics. (1905-1956)

993. ☺ **"I've discovered a way to stay friends forever. There's really nothing to it. I simply tell you what to do and you do it!"**

Silverstein, Shel – a poet, singer-songwriter, cartoonist, and author of children's books. (1930-1999)

994. **"Be careful the environment you choose for it will shape you; be careful the friends you choose for you will become like them."**

Stone, W. Clement – a successful businessman, philanthropist, and self-help book author. He was a high school dropout and a rags-to-riches success story. In 1919, he created the Combined Insurance Company of America, which had more than $1 billion in assets by 1979. (1902-2002)

995. **"Teamwork is what makes common people capable of uncommon results."**

Summitt, Pat – the University of Tennessee women's basketball coach who won eight National Championships and two Olympic gold medals. She retired at age 59 after being diagnosed with Alzheimer's. She ranked #11, and the only woman, on the *Sporting News*' list of the "50 Greatest Coaches of All Time." (1952-2016)

996. **"To love someone is to show to them their beauty, their worth and their importance."**

Vanier, Jean – a Canadian Catholic philosopher, theologian, and humanitarian who works with people with developmental disabilities in countries throughout the world. He has authored 30 books on religion, disability, normality, success, and tolerance. Vanier makes his home in the L'Arche community in France. (1928-)

997. **"Relationships are all there is. Everything in the universe only exists because it is in relationship to everything else. Nothing exists in isolation. We have to stop pretending we are individuals that can go it alone."**

Wheatley, Margaret – a writer and management consultant on organizational behavior. She has worked all over the world in a wide variety of organizations and has developed an approach that opposes, in her words, "highly controlled mechanistic systems that only create robotic behaviors." (1944-)

998. "Expand your universe one person at a time."

White, M. J. – a worksite health promotion professional, writer, and speaker. He is the creator of Lean Wellness – an approach to transforming lifestyle behaviors at work through continuous improvement in body, mind, and spirit. (1957-)

999. ☺ "Assumptions are the termites of relationships."

Winkler, Henry – an actor, director, and author who is best known for his role as Arthur Fonzarelli in the 1970s sitcom *Happy Days*. (1945-)

1000. ☺ "The best mirror is an old friend."

Zarlenga, Peter – attributed to a Peter Nivio Zarlenga who is believed to have been a poet and author. He is given credit for creating the Flight Organization for Individual Achievement, and authoring *The Orator*, *The Immortal Light of Genius* and *The Love Song*. (1943-2007)

M. J. White

ABOUT THE AUTHOR

M. J. White is a passionate promoter of healthy lifestyle behaviors in the workplace. He founded **WELL Street** in 2007 to assist organizations with worksite health promotion. His **MEDSS** (**M**ove More, **E**at and **D**rink Healthy, **D**on't Use Tobacco, **S**leep Well and **S**tress Less) prescription for a healthy lifestyle provides a simple and effective way to change individual behaviors. His **Lean Wellness** approach to worksite culture change, based on Lean Manufacturing principles that encourage ongoing learning and continuous improvement, is an effective and affordable way to change organizational behaviors.

M. J. has advanced degrees in both education and business. His education background includes teaching, consulting, and school administration. His business experience includes sales and marketing, sales management, and business development. He lives in Chicago and works for Activate Healthcare, a leader in employer-sponsored primary care clinics, where he assists organizations with implementing primary care clinics and creating healthy worksite cultures. His **Lean Wellness Blog and Quotes** has provided inspiring quotes and messages every day since early 2015.

Contact Information

Email:	mjwhite@leanwellness.us
Website:	https://www.leanwellness.us
Facebook:	https://www.facebook.com/leanwellness.usa
Twitter:	https://twitter.com/leanwellness_us
Instagram:	https://www.instagram.com/sparks_of_motivation
Pinterest:	https://www.pinterest.com/sparks_of_motivation

INDEX OF AUTHORS AND SOURCES

Author/Source	Quote Number(s)
Socrates	575
Sophocles	715
Soup, Dr. Cuthbert	507
Spanish Proverb	672
Spiker, Ted	263
Spurgeon, Charles	508 & 905
Spurlock, Morgan	305
Stanley, Edward	174
Starr, Ringo	954
Steinbeck, John	339
Stern, Gil	867
Sternin, Jerry	447
Stevens, Connie	906
Stevenson II, Adlai E.	51 & 837
Stevenson, Robert Louis	944
Stone, W. Clement	886 & 994
Stoppard, Tom	408 & 465
Strait, C. Neil	766
Streep, Meryl	385
Streisand, Barbra	52
Summitt, Pat	386 & 995
SunWolf, Dr.	838
Suzuki, David	175 & 868
Swami Satchidananda	509
Sweeney Paul	368
Sweringen, Terri	869
Swindoll, Chuck	409
Symon, Michael	264
Szent-Gyorgyi, Albert	640
Tagore, Rabindranath	800

M. J. White

INDEX OF HEALTHY HUMOR QUOTES

HABITS

THE BODY (Aging)

THE BODY (Body & Health)

THE BODY (Exercise & Fitness)

THE BODY (Food & Nutrition)

THE BODY (Health Care)

THE BODY (Healthy Lifestyle)

THE BODY (Prevention & Self-care)

THE BODY (Sleep)

THE BODY (Weight Management)

THE MIND (Achievement & Success)

THE MIND (Attitude & Enthusiasm)

THE MIND (Challenges, Change & Choices)

THE MIND (Community & Culture)

THE MIND (Confidence & Courage)

THE MIND (Distractions)

THE MIND (Effort & Willpower)

THE MIND (Experience, Future & Past)

THE MIND (Financial Wellbeing)

THE MIND (Focus & Mindfulness)

THE MIND (Fun, Humor & Laughter)

THE MIND (Goals & Motivation)

THE MIND (Leadership & Responsibility)

THE MIND (Learning, Reading & Wisdom)

THE MIND (Mind, Speech & Thoughts)

THE MIND (Productivity & Teamwork)

THE MIND (Relaxation & Stress Management)

THE MIND (Self-awareness & Time)

THE MIND (Work)

THE SPIRIT (Beauty, Creativity & Individuality)

THE SPIRIT (Belief & Convictions)

THE SPIRIT (Character, Courtesy & Goodness)

THE SPIRIT (Charity & Kindness)

THE SPIRIT (Contentment, Patience & Peace)

THE SPIRIT (Emotions, Energy & Vitality)

THE SPIRIT (Encouragement & Support)

THE SPIRIT (Environment & Nature)

THE SPIRIT (Gratitude)

THE SPIRIT (Happiness & Joy)

THE SPIRIT (Meditation, Prayer & Reflection)

THE SPIRIT (Pets)

THE SPIRIT (Relationships)